I AM WOMAN

Our Journeys to Health,
Happiness and Harmony

Shelena C. Lalji M.D.

ISBN: 146117290X
ISBN-13: 9781461172901
Library of Congress Control Number: 2011907695
CreateSpace, North Charleston, South Carolina

Shelena Lalji, MD, F.A.C.O.G.
Medical Director, Dr. Shel Wellness and Medical Spa
1437 Highway 6
Suite 100
Sugar Land, Texas 77478
281-313-SHEL
Website: www.drshel.com
E-mail: info@drshel.com
Twitter: @drshel
LinkedIn: www.linkedin.com/in/drshel
Facebook: www.facebook.com/drshel
YouTube: www.youtube.com/drshelmedspa
Blog: www.drshel.net/blog

CONTENTS

*All patient stories are their own experiences in their own words.
To protect their privacies, their names have been changed.

DEDICATION

To my brother, Akbar Charania. You lived too few years and joined God at the young age of 25. You are dearly missed by all of us you left behind. Thank you for the 25 beautiful and memorable years. We thank God for blessing our family with you.

ACKNOWLEDGEMENTS

I would like to first and foremost thank every one of my patients who put her health and her trust in my hands. All of you have taught me so much over the years about compassion and appreciation. A special thanks to you incredible people who have shared your stories and experiences for others to learn from. Thank you for generously giving your time, energy and talents to make this happen. This book would not have been possible without you and your transforming stories. Each of you has inspired my journey to make a difference in people's lives—be it big or small. For this, I want to say a big, heartfelt, and sincere Thank you!

Next, I would like to thank my team of devoted and wonderful women with whom I work daily, and who assist me in caring for our patients and to help them live their best lives possible. You all help me to keep our patients healthy, empowered and balanced. A special thanks to Jennifer Hill Robenault for all her assistance with the book and to Dana Vogenthaler for always being by my side as we made the exciting journey for this book. Thank you!

For us to accomplish anything of true value, we need support—from our partner, our family, our friends, and other women who have gone through, or are going through, the same physical challenges that we are. I could not have pursued this healing journey without these extraordinary people in my life. Allow me to introduce you to a few of them:

First of all, my husband Dr. Ayeez Lalji. He has over the past fourteen years been my best friend, confidante, supporter, and biggest source of inspiration for me to follow my dreams, whatever they may be. I am truly blessed to have him in my life. My inner circle consists of Ayeez and our two wonderful children—our ten-year-old daughter, Zoe, and our seven-year-old son, Zade. I feel boundless gratitude for the blessings of my children and my extraordinary husband. We share the deep bond of family, but it's more than that, they make me laugh, inspire me, comfort me, and bring me back to my true self on a daily basis. With them, I dive deep into experiencing the most important aspect of human life: love. The joy that we share gives me strength, purpose, and a sense of well-being that is truly indescribable. My darlings, I thank you far more than words can say

Second, my two mothers: my birth mother, Nazline–the one who gave birth to me, raised me, taught me the values I live by every day, made me the woman I am today, and showed me how to always give back and help those in need. And my mother-in-law, Gulshen, who supports me daily in keeping our home and family together and gives me love and support so I can help my patients and fellow women tirelessly. Thank you both!

Third, my father, Firoz, for teaching me the values I live by, giving me the work ethic that gets me through my hectic schedules, and always giving me the encouragement "to do the right thing". He has been a role model of hard work and unflinching commitment to one's goals. Thanks to my brother, Farid, who has always demonstrated strength, perseverance and a good sense of humor. I still remember the days we used to play as kids and will always cherish them. Also, my father-in-law, Amir, for being a kind and gentle soul.

Fourth, my two best friends and sisters, Nadiya and Shirin. They are the mirrors that always reflect the truth about me. They support me tirelessly and are always there for me . . . no matter the day or time. We have shared laughter, happiness, secrets, as well as our sorrows both as children and adults . . . and we have grown stronger by the year. Thank you both, to my soul sisters!

Next, my two new sisters, Sheniz and Ezmin (my sisters-in-law). Thank you for being so giving and caring and extending your love to me since we became family.

Finally, to all my dear girlfriends and colleagues with whom I have grown up with, shared happiness and tears as fellow women… you all have taught me about the bonds that women have and absolutely, undoubtedly need in their lives. Thanks to you all!

I am grateful for the experiences I have had throughout the course of my career in medicine. I feel deeply satisfied knowing that I have been blessed with the ability to positively change people's lives. My hope is that I continue to learn, to share, and to connect with women who need new information about the wonders of their bodies, and how they can be improved or healed. In this book, I want to share extraordinary knowledge I have gained for solving this evolutionary problem. My hope is that we can all live fuller, richer, happier lives in every phase of our time on this earth . . . in mind, body, and spirit. Cheers to you all!

INTRODUCTION

*W*e are all constantly evolving in life. That is a good thing. Being stagnant by definition keeps us from growing. One of my major evolutions was going from traditional to integrative medicine. Integrative medicine, contrary to popular belief, is based upon scientific facts, which are backed by insurmountable studies. The practice and mastery of integrative medicine delicately combines the laws and principles of traditional medicine that are needed to understand the body biologically, along with the strong desire to treat patients as unique individuals, not case studies. It revolves around treating the complete body, not simply its parts, which at times leads us to running around to different physicians who specialize in treating their specialized systems.

Practitioners who provide integrative treatments can spend 5 to10 times more time getting to know their patients' symptoms, history, goals and emotional well-being as it relates to their health. This approach allows the patient to be viewed as a completely "new" challenge. This typically results in the lack of "cookie-cutter" treatments, which unfortunately, most of us have been subjected to at some point in regards to our health care. Integrative medicine utilizes individualized care by the physician, specialized diagnostic testing, and natural alternatives to treat root causes of symptoms. Lifestyle modifications and compliance from the patient are also essential parts.

This type of medicine has noticed great strides in the direction of preventive care as people are searching for more options that are in harmony with their bodies and beliefs. The focus of these types of treatments is based upon each unique patient's interest, not the interest of insurance companies or pharmaceutical companies. When you decide to make the decision to choose this type of care, you may be deterred by many people, but once they notice the positive impact it has had on your life they will become more supportive and likely seek it for themselves. If my wishes came true...everyone would be inspired to educate themselves on the countless benefits of moving in the direction of natural care, as opposed to more traditional modalities. As with everything...education is key, which is why I took the time to write this book for you.

My shift into integrative medicine was one that took over 10 years. After practicing as a Board Certified Ob/Gyn for many years, I felt a deep-seated calling to treat women in a way I felt was destined for me. It was the result of my upbringing, my values, and my experience with thousands of women suffering from life changing symptoms that were treated based on those symptoms alone...not the cause of their symptoms.

I knew at a young age that I wanted to be an Ob/Gyn to ultimately help women by being their strongest advocate and supporter for a life full of health and vitality. The more I became immersed in my professional practice, the further I got from my values and ultimate vision. I knew I had to change. I began educating myself and endlessly studied as I looked for the true answers to my patients' concerns. Once the answers were realized, it didn't take me long to understand I could do so much more for my patients while still practicing medicine the way I *wanted* to, and the way they *needed* me to.

For this book, nine women, from my current integrative practice, graciously agreed (and were excited) to share their stories, told in their own words, to help women everywhere know that they are not alone in the struggles they may be having. They too believed that your struggles do not have to be written off as "part of the natural aging process", "too much stress", "not enough sleep", or any other excuse that we like to believe to help ourselves feel better about our current state of health. An unhealthy state does not have to only relate to cancer, high blood pressure and cholesterol, diabetes, or any other image relating to disease that may come to mind. But, the truth is, if your current symptoms aren't treated in the appropriate way, your body can begin to experience unhealthy inflammation, which eventually does lead to a compromised state of health, and ultimately, disease.

This is what I explain to my patients, not with the intent to scare them, but instead to empower them to stand up and take control of their state of health, be it physical, psychological, emotional, or spiritual. If we are lacking in any of these areas of health, we are lacking balance. I want you to be informed and inspired by my patients' stories so you too can regain your balance in whatever areas are suited to your needs. I encourage you to use the sections designated for your notes after each story to discover what areas you would like to improve in your life and what steps to take to reach your goals of *Health, Happiness, and Harmony.*

PART ONE:

The Journey Begins

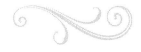

"Life has no limitations,
except the ones you make"

LES BROWN

CHAPTER 1:
THE CHALLENGES FACING WOMEN TODAY

"For every promise you make to others,
keep one to yourself"

SARAH BAN BREATHNACH

*A*s a doctor, I tend to dispense a lot of advice. That's what I am trained to do, and that's what my patients ask of me. We each have our roles. I have my diplomas, my credentials, and my will to serve. I have compassion in my heart, and an earnest and deep-seated need to help people be unafraid and to live their lives to the absolute fullest. I want my patients to use the information I share with them to become strong, empowered, and even brave. This may sound a bit melodramatic, but I request for you to open your mind and heart to very real new possibilities within close reach.

Women come to me with symptoms. Sometimes the symptoms are grave, but the patient is not fearful. Sometimes the symptoms are mild, but the patient is swallowed in anxiety. Suffice it to say, a woman's emotions regarding her physical state are unique and highly complex. Our bodies tell the outward stories of our lives. They can show how we really feel about ourselves and if the world has been harsh to us. Our bodies reveal how hard we work or how little time we have to tend to our own needs. A woman's body can bear many characteristics from critical experiences and choices in her life—a scar from a Cesarean section, hunched shoulders from working long hours at a computer, extra weight from eating for comfort or out of loneliness. Then there are the scars of abuse, neglect, and depression. Yes, our bodies tell incredible stories of what we've been through and where we've been.

So, patients come to me for cures, solutions, and hope. In the beginning of my career, I was like most physicians— I was the expert, the educated one. Patients needed to do what I recommended, because after all, I was the doctor. I have to admit that I did have a few colleagues who mutated these qualities into sheer arrogance. They maintained an emotional distance from patients, and held up their abilities to do so like trophies or awards. I tried to keep myself grounded, and always gravitated toward wanting to know the full story behind each and every person I treated. Back then, I was still the teacher, and the patient was still the student. Once I started to practice, that relationship began to evolve.

I wish I could write an eloquent and heroic account of when I discovered with certainty that the way I had been taught to practice medicine was not in my patients' best interests. No one patient or one dramatic emergency room experience left me so angry or devastated that I decided to go off on my own and redefine what medicine was to me, telling me that I did not want to participate in a field that is historically steeped in the avoidance and anticipation of death. No, it was a gradual process that spanned over a few years. I felt as though I was in the center of the parable that states when a frog is thrown into a boiling pot of water, it jumps out; but when it is thrown into a cool pot of water and heated gradually, before it is any the wiser, it has been boiled to death. The story is a metaphor for people's complacency. I did not want to be that frog!

At a certain point, I simply had to come clean with myself about what I truly believed the practice of healing to be. Healing is a sacred partnership between one who wants to help and the recipient of that help or assistance. I realized one absolute truth…we are all healers. Every time we look someone in the eye who is in the throes of sorrow, and we offer him or her a kind word or a helping hand, we are healers. This philosophy reminds me of the powerful soliloquy that Robin Williams delivers at the end of the film *Patch Adams*. Patch Adams was an actual medical student in the 1970s who desperately wanted to become a physician. He possessed deep compassion for his patients, and was known for making personal connections with them. He often used humor and other unorthodox methods to help improve the lives of his patients. This is his speech imploring the board of the medical school to allow him to graduate. I identified with the story of this unique doctor. In the film, Patch Adams sums up most eloquently what I believe about the sacred contract between a doctor and patient:

Now, I've sat in your schools and heard people lecture on transference and professional distance. Transference is inevitable, sir. Every human being has an impact on another. Why don't we want that in a patient/doctor relationship? That's why I've listened to your teachings, and I believe they're wrong. A doctor's mission should be not just to prevent death but also to improve the quality of life. That's why when you treat a disease, you win, you lose; however, when you treat a person, I guarantee you, you win, no matter what the outcome. Now here today, this room is full of medical students. [He turns to the students.] Don't let them anesthetize you. Don't let them numb you out to the miracle of life. Always live in awe of the glorious mechanism of the human body. Let that be the focus of your studies and not a quest for grades, which will give you no idea what kind of doctor you will become. Don't wait till you're on the ward to get your humanity back. Start your interviewing skills. Start talking to strangers. Talk to your friends, talk to wrong numbers, everyone. . . . Sir, I want to be a doctor with all my heart. I wanted to become a doctor so I could serve others . . . and because of that I've lost everything . . . but I've also gained everything. I've shared the lives of patients and staff members at the hospital. I've laughed with them. I've cried with them. This is what I want to do with my life.

I had to keep true to myself, I wanted to be a healer, and I wanted to help women overcome the troublesome physiological repercussions of time spent away from their true selves. I can look into a woman's eyes and see the most beautiful creature in the world just waiting to reclaim what is hers—a life of vitality, strength, love, and beauty. We all deserve to lead the life that was intended for us. But we worry about the "what if's." As a result, our lives become crippled with anxiety and fear about what will happen if we actually take time for ourselves. This manner of thinking foretells the beginning of the end of a fulfilling life for many women.

I spent a lot of time considering the title of this book. The topic of women's health is vast, despite the surprisingly deficient amount of research that has been done regarding the unique physical, hormonal, and psychological issues that women face daily. I considered calling this book *A Woman's Wake-Up Call,* which seemed very appropriate on some level. Women need to wake up to the benefits of the information and resources available to them that could vastly improve the quality of their lives on every level. Unfortunately, tracking down the facts can still be something like a treasure hunt. Women must be extremely proactive in understanding that they are not alone and they are not losing their minds when they experience specific symptoms; fortunately, help truly is available, albeit difficult to find at times

I also decided, with great consideration, not to focus on the word "menopause," simply because this word tends to instill a lot of confusion and concern in many women. As you read through the remarkable true stories in this book, you will understand why women from ages thirty-four to fifty-eight chose to share their personal battles with symptoms that left them dejected and hopeless. Some of them simply had no idea that they were peri-menopausal or postmenopausal. The word "menopause" conjures up ideas of hot flashes, night sweats, and moody women past their reproductive years. But complications from hormonal imbalances can strike at any age—even in women as young as thirty. I would like to leave the menopause conversation for those who have come before me, and who have done an excellent and thorough job of explaining the complexities and challenges of the menopausal woman. Through this book, however, I want to encourage my fellow women to do five important things:

1. **Get help.** If you are not feeling like yourself, find a board-certified physician who understands the "whole patient" and who has the skills and knowledge to treat you holistically.

2. **Become your own advocate.** If something does not feel right, don't give up until you find a treatment protocol that works for you. Only you can determine the effectiveness of treatment practices for you.

3. **Get educated.** Spend time understanding the profound links between your body, mind, and spirit. The ultimate goal is to feel aligned in these three areas for optimal health and well-being.

4. **Share information.** Tell your story about overcoming your health issues by becoming hormonally and nutritionally balanced to others. Encourage your sisters, mothers, friends, and aunts to look beyond traditional medicine in addressing health concerns.

5. **Celebrate your life.** Once your body is in balance and you are on your way there, enjoy and celebrate your life! Live it to its fullest, and be a role model of Health, Happiness, and Harmony to the other women in your life.

The urgency of the situation cannot be ignored. After being engrossed in women's health for the last seventeen years, I feel a responsibility and am blessed to be in a unique position to reveal the disturbing trends in women's health that keep surfacing over and over again. Nearly every patient who walks through my doors has a variation of the same list of complaints: **weight gain, mood swings, depression, fatigue, sleep disruptions, hair loss, low libido (sex drive), anxiety, body aches, and many more symptoms that are far too common and far too often overlooked**. Simply put, they feel exhausted, overwhelmed, and not so sexy. They feel as though they are aging rapidly, through a process that is out of their control. In short, the majority of the women who come to me have confided, *"I just don't feel like myself anymore."*

For some women, the latest information on women's health and wellness may very well save their lives. Yes, it is *that* important. Understanding your body, your hormones, the aging process, and the logistics of your libido can profoundly and forever alter your life for the better. It can relieve you from a vicious cycle of fatigue, depression, anxiety, and perpetual weight gain. On a deeper level, taking control of your wellness may even save your marriage, improve your relationships with family and friends, and create a model of health and well-being that can become a life-altering foundation for the future health of your children or any young person who looks up to you. I genuinely believe it is my job to forge a new path that provides gentle, reassuring guidance. This is a huge responsibility and endeavor that I take very seriously. I also take great pride and joy in being able to somehow, on some small level, help my fellow women. So, yes, perhaps the whole "wake-up call" notion may seem a bit harsh, but it certainly rings true for most women.

Why did I finally decide to call this book *I Am Woman*? It's simple. Women are hard enough on themselves already. In many ways, we really are our own worst enemies. Many of us would never treat a child, a friend, or any loved one the way we often treat ourselves. I am committed to helping women reclaim themselves, and to get in touch with the women within by pulling back the curtain on what the larger medical community is really doing (or not doing) about the rampant symptoms that are literally plaguing women in this country and around the world. In spiritual terms, Buddhists would encourage women to seek their "true selves." In other religious terms, people are encouraged to "know thyself." Regardless of your spiritual leaning, nothing is more human, more essential, more beautiful, or more important than going fearlessly in the direction of understanding the divine connection between your body, mind, and spirit. It is a very human journey to health, happiness, and harmony, and I feel very privileged to be able to use my professional training to help women tackle this emotional issue of regaining control of their bodies so they can ultimately achieve wellness.

The phrase *"I Am Woman"* creates an image for all women to follow and feel empowered to stand up for themselves. A strong and empowered woman is someone who decides, against all of society's pressures, insistence, and attempts to condition, that living authentically and truthfully in every aspect of her life takes precedence over all else. Women are told to do, to be, to act, to look, to think, and to feel differently—more often than not—in ways that are counter to our natural state of being and living. Our natural state is one of joy, freedom, acceptance, peace, happiness, and contentment—even during times of extreme adversity. It's been said many times that we cannot control what happens to us. However, we absolutely can control how we react to any circumstance or situation. We can choose how to feel and how to behave. This ability is yet another extraordinary byproduct of being human. We get to decide whether to listen to our bodies, our hearts, our feelings, and our gut instincts. We can abide by the strong inner wisdom that we all possess, or we can ignore it and continue to climb a very steep and difficult path toward that elusive state of happiness.

So many women feel they must be in total control at all times to fulfill a certain destiny or to remain steadfast on a life path they wholeheartedly believe will lead them to a sense of freedom and joy. But I believe there is something to be said for the act of letting go and allowing the universe, other people, and the mystery of life to unfold in unexpected ways. As a physician, I completely understand the dynamics of the five senses: sight, sound, taste, touch, and smell. But we also have a sixth sense—our intuition or, as some people describe it, that small, still voice that never lies to us, never deceives us, and never asks us to harm ourselves or others.

In other words, when we manage to appreciate life's gifts and the extraordinary ways that the universe systematically and consistently provides for our needs, we find ourselves in a state of health, balance, and overall well-being. Women want to feel in control, and we want balance in our lives. For me, achieving balance between my professional and personal life is most challenging. I urge you to seek support systems that will allow you to find or maintain that balance by stepping in when you need them to. In my case, my two strongest supporters are my sweet, darling husband, Ayeez, who himself is a busy dentist and entrepreneur but still makes time to do so much for our children; and my highly giving and loving mother-in-law, Gulshen, who always helps me with my children when I need her. I attain balance because of supporters like them, and so can you!

Women have been told over and over again that they can gain this state of control in their lives by creating balance, and everyone has different methods to achieve it. Eat less. Exercise more. Get more rest. Increase intake of fruits and vegetables. Walk. Run. Swim. Do yoga. Think happier thoughts. Pray. Relax. Read certain books. In other words, *you* must be in charge of your health. Only *you* can change your life. Well, this goal is not as simple as it may seem. Yes, you are in charge of making decisions about a great many things. But at a certain point, a physiological reality kicks in for all of us and we may feel very out of control because of these physical and hormonal changes. I'm here to share many patients' stories to demonstrate the profound link between your hormones and your body to help you become a lifelong advocate for your own health.

I had been living in Georgia for more than sixteen years, from 1981 to 1997—high school, college, medical school, and residency. It was a wonderful time in my life. After I completed my residency, I knew I wanted to start my own OB-GYN practice as a solo practitioner, which seemed absolutely crazy to many of my colleagues and friends. But I came from a family of entrepreneurs, and I knew I wanted to be successful while serving women on my own terms. Having completed my traditional medical training, I had experienced firsthand the dysfunction of the typical patient/doctor relationship.

Medical students are continually encouraged to observe patients in an emotionally distant way. They are taught that this attitude is an act of professionalism and objectivity as well as a crucial practice for emotional self-preservation. In emergency situations, doctors are compelled to make tough decisions about a patient's treatment. When a life is on the line, they are taught to have nerves of steel and to focus on the body as an object, 100 percent. This aspect of practicing medicine always felt counter to what I felt about my patients' care. I believed that compassion was a driving motivator in why I chose this profession, so to be discouraged from personally connecting with my patients seemed unnecessary and quite heartbreaking. It was impossible for me to look into someone's eyes and to not try to understand what that person's life might be like and how his or her health may have been compromised due to things beyond mere genetics or life choices. I knew that, so many times, my patients were at the mercy of their bodies, which their and others' decisions had likely treated poorly.

I have never felt compelled to judge a woman who is overweight and suffering from complications with diabetes, for example. I could always imagine that she may have experienced a difficult childhood, poor role models, low self-esteem, or maybe even abuse or addiction. My interactions with early patients were some of the most intimate and authentic exchanges with people I have ever had. So it was imperative to me, as I went out on my own, that I create a practice and culture of treating women that truly reflected my own values, not just as a doctor but as a person. How could I teach my patients to face themselves and to travel that harrowing path to living with integrity if I did not do the same?

I had to be very honest with myself and my treatment style. My goals as a physician started to become much clearer as a steady stream of irritable, depressed, apathetic, fatigued women came to seek help after visiting dozens of "traditional" doctors. I knew they needed the time and space to discuss their histories, to divulge their fears, and even to shed a few tears. (I always keep two tissue boxes within reach in my office—one for my patients and, at times, one for me.) I learn things in my first thirty-minute conversation with a patient that a traditional doctor might miss and that could seriously alter a treatment course. Physicians are trained to throw antidepressants at a problem instead of carefully building a portrait of a woman who may, for example, be suffering from severe adrenal fatigue.

So, as you read this book, you will learn about common conditions and treatments that are changing the way women are being healed today. You'll read personal stories about women who have overcome common issues, including hormone imbalances, severe stress, loss of sex drive, hair loss, depression, weight gain, fatigue, sleep disorders, and much more. But, most importantly, you will know—beyond a shadow of a doubt—that you are not alone. You will understand how to become an advocate for your own health and how to live as an active and enthusiastic champion of a new era in women's health. Congratulations.

My Challenges

What are your personal challenges that

you would like to overcome?

_____
_____
_____
_____
_____
_____
_____
_____
_____
_____
_____
_____
_____
_____
_____
_____
_____
_____
_____
_____
_____
_____
_____
_____
_____
_____

CHAPTER 2:
FROM OB/GYN TO INTEGRATIVE
PRACTITIONER & HEALER

"People will forget what you said,
people will forget what you did,
but people will never forget
how you made them feel"

MAYA ANGELOU

I became a doctor to heal people. What I learned after many years of having an OB-GYN practice treating women from all socioeconomic backgrounds, age groups, and ethnicities, is that medicine is under siege. It has evolved into an industry that cannot and does not treat the whole human being. Doctors treat the body and the symptoms, but we unfortunately ignore the heart and mind that complete this divine map of being. We have become trapped in a web of hierarchies, protocols, and profits. We have ceased to provide sincere, honest treatment for those who need it in exchange for retrofitting our own needs and lives into a system that is inherently flawed and tragically broken. At this stage in the game, doctors are rarely permitted to provide high-quality, low-cost health care to the people who need it most. And patients, trapped by the extraordinary expense of health care, may only seek attention when symptoms can no longer be ignored. This ineffective dynamic does not support prevention and a well-being mind-set. As a society, we are caught up in an emergency and reactive culture that focuses on saving rather than on preventing or healing.

Although this information may not be news, I feel it is important that I, as a physician, stand and be counted as a medical professional who deeply desires to treat the whole person: body, mind, and spirit. It's imperative that individuals who are expertly trained in medicine publicly and consistently acknowledge the profound link between all parts of the human self.

I am grateful that integrative medicine is becoming more and more accepted among mainstream patients. We see studies every day that tell us yoga, acupuncture, massage, and meditation can all promote health and well-being. These practices are now solidly included in the popular Western lexicon, thus affording new generations an opportunity to seamlessly integrate Eastern modalities into their visions of health maintenance and overall well-being. This broader approach is great news for patients, but many of these practices may seem like voodoo to the traditional medical establishment that still depends on symptom-based treatment.

My Indian culture and my family have deeply formed how I view my patients, my practice, and my life. My Indian background includes a deep sense of family obligation and devotion to children, as exists in most cultures. But coming from an impoverished nation where I routinely witnessed a lack of health care and resources for women and children left a profound and indelible mark on my psyche. My desire to help people and to become an OB-GYN was born there. Being surrounded by people who were affected by poverty and limited opportunities, I always felt the need to compensate for what they did not have. I had been able to do this to a certain degree by practicing as a traditional Ob/Gyn, but eventually I hit a roadblock.

It was rewarding and exciting in the beginning. But the reality of the health-care system soon set in. I had been feeling a little empty about my Ob/Gyn practice, believing that I could and should be doing more to help the women who were desperate to find answers to their varied health concerns. The focus of my traditional work was delivering babies, providing prenatal care, and treating women's reproductive health. But more and more, my patients complained of feeling "off" or not understanding simply how or why their bodies were changing over time. Additionally, I was not fully prepared during my many years of education for the sheer number of women who suffer psychologically and emotionally. I am not a therapist, psychiatrist, or a social worker, but as a physician I have extensive knowledge of the relationship between depression, hormones, and the general state of lethargy or "dullness" that women experience every day. I became very aware that a serious, ongoing lack of emotional support and self-esteem could wreak havoc on a woman's body and psyche. As depression deepens, synapses in the brain radically change, and chemicals within the body dramatically begin to work against you. At that point, it becomes more and more difficult to heal from that state without serious psychological and medical intervention. But I never imagined that one of my closest friends would suffer so tragically.

Maya's Story: Tragic Loss for Me, More Determination for My Mission

Does losing someone ever make sense? I lost my brother at a young age, so you would think I would be prepared for this, but I wasn't. Inside and out, Maya was one of the most beautiful women I ever had the honor to call my friend. In fact, she was my best friend. She stood tall and lean and possessed remarkable authenticity and poise. I thought she was like a living goddess, and I trusted her with the secrets of my life. I hope everyone has the privilege of having a soul friend like Maya. She was a brilliant doctor with a very reputable medical group in Atlanta. She was a beloved colleague to so many people—an amazing woman who any man in the world would have been fortunate to have in his life. She was exceptionally successful, she looked sensational, and she had a very witty sense of humor. Women wanted to be her, or at least be close enough to her to have a bit of Maya's magic rub off on them.

But Maya had one extremely serious problem—she was married to an emotionally abusive man. Maya's husband wanted an independent life and was not emotionally ready to be committed to anyone—even if she happened to be one of the most stunning, intelligent, kind, and amazing women he would ever have the good fortune to meet in this lifetime.

Over time, Maya became increasingly distraught, because the man she loved simply did not value her. He was an eighteen-year-old in a thirty-year-old man's body. He was selfish, thoughtless, and unkind. Most children are not as emotionally reckless as this man was. It was a complete mystery to me why Maya would marry such an emotionally unavailable person. Any man would have been lucky to have her. But for reasons that have never become clear to me, Maya settled. It was her extreme misfortune that she happened to fall in love with this person. But what I learned from their relationship is that you absolutely cannot or should not attempt to control the people around you. Whether it's your mother, father, sister, brother, spouse, friend, or child, the only person you have any power over is you. How you react to dysfunctional people is the only thing you have any emotional jurisdiction over at any given moment. You cannot let others dictate how you feel about yourself, your life, or your future. Unfortunately, a lot of women choose not to exercise or to accept that control. It was heartbreaking for me to see that Maya could not recognize her own power.

My sister and I were essentially Maya's family for many years. We were her sisters, not by blood but by soul. When my sister got engaged, perhaps my sister's joy made Maya realize what she was missing in her own life. We'll never really know. What we know now is that Maya was in a very, very dark place. It's a mind-set I have never experienced, and I pray that no one in my life or in my care will ever have to endure it.

One week before my sister's engagement party, Maya bought a gun, put it to her head, and shot herself. We were absolutely devastated. It is rare for a woman to commit suicide in this manner, but Maya was a focused person, and when she put her mind to something, she did it. The tragic irony of this otherwise-positive personality trait was not lost on anyone who deeply loved her. Why couldn't she have used that strength and determination to leave her marriage, to seek counseling, and to restore herself to who she really was? In the end, perhaps she had gone too far into that dark place, and no one could reach her. She was lost forever.

When Maya died, my mission in life began to slowly change. I began to realize that I had to do everything in my power to prevent another woman from killing herself because of such a serious lack of self-esteem. I see so many women who take care of their husbands and their children and go through life earning a living and taking care of business. Then the day arrives when everything comes to a head, and suddenly a sense of loss, confusion, and despair sets in. They start to ask themselves, "Who am I?" and "What happened to me?" and "Is this all there is?" They are completely unaware of the fact that they have quickly spiraled downward into that dangerous, dark place that took Maya's life. They don't notice how bad things have gotten until they hit rock bottom. And when they look up, they can't even see the light. It is completely dark, and imposing, scary walls of despair and isolation surround them. How do they climb out? For Maya, it was too late. But my goal is to prevent women from falling into that desperate, dangerous, and dark hole in the first place.

I began to tell Maya's story to patients. I started to understand that sharing her story was not only therapeutic to the women who came to see me but was healing for me as well. It was then that I realized that the doctor/patient relationship had a reciprocal nature that I had not acknowledged before. I had patients hugging me and extending their compassion and kindness to me in such extraordinary ways that I began to understand the power of women coming together as peers and friends to heal and to change lives.

I don't know if I can ever really reconcile what happened to Maya. To this day, I still feel as though I could have done something to prevent it. But I know that if I can help heal other women from the inside out, I'll be paying an honest and heartfelt tribute to my beautiful friend. I miss her.

As a spiritual woman, I believe God has a profound and important purpose for my life and for that of everyone around me. Our ability to serve others matches our ability to serve God and the evolution of consciousness on this planet. So, today, I am a doctor, wife, mother, sister, daughter, friend, and woman. I am like so many women in the United States, trying daily to understand how to live my best possible life while also acting in conscious and loving service to my family and to my community. In all truth, I have the benefit of knowing how to remain clear and focused in how my life operates, because I intimately understand our power, as well as our vulnerabilities, as human beings.

Simply put, we can all make a big difference, even with a minute act. It is infinitely easier to dream big and to have the energy and momentum to execute those dreams when your body supports you. However, you don't have to be a weight lifter or a model or even good at a sport. You just have to make a commitment to be in tune with who you really are at any given moment. What are you feeling? What is your body feeling? Can you allow yourself to feel all these complicated feelings and sensations in your body, your heart, and your mind long enough to understand where you are strong and where you are weak? Or will you continue to do everything in your power to mask these feelings and put off, for yet another day, the important and divine work of knowing yourself?

I am spiritual, but I am also a scientist. I believe in the connection between divine gifts and hard facts. In my worldview, no conflict exists between what I see under a microscope and what I can sense of someone's emotional life. The seen and the unseen, in my view, have always coexisted powerfully.

This isn't the first or the last time you'll hear the message that women simply don't take care of themselves the way they know they should. The excuses are limitless, and an entire self-care industry has emerged specifically around our deep desire to strike that important balance between family, career, other commitments, and self. However far we have come as women, we are still utterly confused about what we need to do to feel better about ourselves and the lives we lead. This is why I chose the work that I do—to help women examine their lives in new ways that keep them healthy, happy, and vibrant.

For most doctors, healing is an art that demystifies and makes quick sense of the intricacies and complexities of the human body under attack, stress, or extreme change. There is the complaint, the consultation, the testing, the diagnosis, and the treatment. We are at war with a disease, an injury, or a mysterious set of symptoms. We are problem solvers, detectives, scientists, engineers, sculptors . . . and sometimes just incredibly lucky. We are, above all, human beings. This last description is most important to me as a healer—to be human.

My Passions

Are you going in the direction of your passion?

How can you tap into the "true you"?

_____
_____
_____
_____
_____
_____
_____
_____
_____
_____
_____
_____
_____
_____
_____
_____
_____
_____
_____
_____
_____
_____
_____
_____
_____
_____
_____

CHAPTER 3:
LOSS . . . A TURNING POINT

"And in the end it's not the years in your life that count.
It's the life in your years"

ABRAHAM LINCOLN

My Loss

I was a twenty year old student at Emory University, living at home, and studying for exams to get into medical school. It was a busy and exciting time in my life. I was very close to my sisters, and we loved our two brothers immensely. My older brother was twenty-five years old, was married, and had two children, ages two-and-a-half years and eight months.

At that time, my brother was running my father's factory in another city and was his right-hand man. My mother would often say that if her five children were the fingers on a hand, my older brother would be the thumb—nothing worked without him. He was our guide and protector. He was strong, hardworking, and loving. To us, he was everything.

In February 1989, my brother had traveled to Atlanta for a family celebration. We were all there, laughing, dancing, and truly having the time of our lives. I remember my brother lifting his 2-½ year old daughter, Shezi, onto his shoulders and dancing. It was a beautiful event. He was scheduled to go back home the next day but decided to extend his stay to spend more time with his family.

During the previous year, my brother had become very spiritual. We had all noticed it but nobody understood why at the time. He routinely woke up to meditate at 4:30 a.m., and he seemed more introspective than usual. My father told us later about a conversation he and my brother had as they pondered the meaning of life. My brother had traveled the world, was married to a loving woman, had two beautiful children, had achieved financial success, and had fulfilled all his dreams. He had asked my father, "Is there anything more to live for?" Of course, my father told him that he was still a young man and had his entire life ahead of him, without thinking much of it.

The night before my brother was to travel back home, he was at the hotel owned by my family helping to take care of some important work. He, my uncle, and my mother were in the hotel lobby when a drunken gunman opened fire without any reason. My uncle was shot in the arm, but my brother managed to escape and run outside. When he realized that our mother was still in the lobby, he ran back inside to protect her and came face to face with the gunman. He was shot five times in the torso and chest, and my mother witnessed the entire scene. Completely hysterical beyond comprehension, she ran to her son, who was bleeding out in front of her very eyes.

I was taking care of my brother's infant son when this was happening, and I remember later learning his time of death. It was at that precise moment that my nephew had begun hysterically wailing and crying. I believe on some spiritual level, that he knew his father had passed away. It was such a heartbreaking and overwhelming experience, one that no family ever believes it will have to suffer through. We had lived such a peaceful and close-knit existence as a family, moving from one country to the next and being each other's closest friends. How would we survive this tragedy?

After the murder, everything changed. My father suffered a heart attack and subsequently had two bypass surgeries. We were all convinced that he would die within a few months of the tragedy. But he came through the experience—we all did. Amid the most tragic experience of my life, I could have easily given up and resorted to a life full of sadness, questions, and distractions away from my destined course. However, just the opposite resulted—my brother's death increased my desire and passion to push forward on my mission to heal and to promote health and happiness in as many patients as possible, just as I was doing for myself and my family as we worked to overcome our loss. I was accepted to Georgetown Medical School in Washington, D.C., but I decided instead to stay at Emory University to be close to my family. I needed them, and they needed me. Together we grieved, shared great memories of my brother, and allowed our sense of strength to prosper just as my brother would have wished.

This experience, like every individual human experience, gave us the ability to change how and what we do with the time we have here on Earth. My mission to become a healer was solidified by my brother's death, and, in turn, I'm proud to have delivered hundreds of babies and to have helped thousands of women improve their health. Ultimately, becoming an OB-GYN was healing for me. I was bringing new life into the world and helping women understand their bodies and appreciate their own lives. I felt a deep connection to my patients, and one of my most satisfying feelings is to make a difference in people's lives on a regular basis.

My Personal Losses

What losses are you dealing with that have impacted

your life? How can you grow from them and

be a positive influence to other people?

_____

_____

_____

_____

_____

_____

_____

_____

_____

_____

_____

_____

_____

_____

_____

_____

_____

_____

_____

_____

_____

_____

_____

_____

_____

CHAPTER 4:
THE CULTURES THAT SHAPED ME

*"Don't be scared to present the "real you" to the world-
authenticity is at the heart of success"*

CIQUI CARTAGENA

I was born in India, and we lived there until I was five years old. Even from such a young age, I retain vivid memories of trips my family and I would take. It was not unusual to see incredible, unbelievable poverty all around us. The sight of children with no limbs or who were blind or extremely ill was something that I could not comprehend. I think anyone who hasn't experienced it firsthand can never fully process the emotional impact of seeing children who do not even have their basic needs met. It's overwhelming. The situation feels completely out of control, ruthless, and sad beyond comprehension. Even as a child, I knew that those children who were constantly begging for money were someone's sons and daughters.

It took me many years to come to terms with what existed around us in the most nonchalant, everyday sort of way. I suppose if you spend your life in India, you make peace with it on some level—you have to. People have to find ways to cope with the brutality of other people's lives. The history there cannot be penetrated just by saying, "Enough! No more children can experience this hardship anymore!" Change happens slowly, and is a result of the passion and commitment of many incredible individuals. I felt very motivated to become a doctor and to achieve a certain amount of success to bring change to causes and people I cared about.

I knew that wherever I was on my life's path, I would feel motivated to help whoever came my way. My work has led me to help women heal their bodies and see their inherent value as human beings. Once women heal themselves, their families and relationships have the foundation to heal and to grow as well. Happy, healthy people find meaning and purpose in life, which inevitably enables them to influence their communities and the causes they care about in untold ways. This work—for my patients and me—is about honoring ourselves and valuing others.

Even today, those memories of India are very sharp. I would later understand that helplessness was the one totally encompassing feeling of being in a third-world country. More than twenty-five million orphans live in India—a total greater than the entire population of the state of Texas. Where does one even begin to make a difference?

During my life, I have felt extremely fortunate to have a present and loving family on my side. They are my strength and my foundation. I knew that I would always have their support and assistance in achieving my personal goals and any dream I could imagine. I do not take this kind of love for granted. It is one of my greatest blessings.

When I was five, my family and I moved to England. When I was ten, we moved to New Jersey. When I was twelve, we made our final move as a family to the place I called home … Atlanta, Georgia. Our constant moving required my entire family to be very close-knit. I grew up with two brothers and two sisters, and we depended on one another implicitly. We were (and had to be) each other's best friends, because we never lived anywhere long enough to make and to sustain long-term friendships until we moved to Atlanta, Georgia.

I had a very happy childhood. My father was a self-made man who created and built his own wealth. I respect and admire him so much for his ability to take risks, to have a vision, and to execute it. He taught us these values, and we live by his example. He followed through on business ideas and made things happen. He had an incredible work ethic and a clear ambition to care for us in the best way possible. Because I had the friendship and companionship of my brothers and sisters, I loved that we lived and traveled around the world. The experience not only gave me a deep appreciation for other cultures and people but made me feel that the world was accessible and open to me at any time. The world was indeed my backyard.

I spent the majority of my childhood in the Atlanta area. My parents owned hotels there, and my siblings and I were expected to be an integral part of the family business. We did everything. I cleaned rooms, checked in guests, did laundry, and eventually handled the bookkeeping. In my family, you were taught to make your own way in life with the support of family, a deep faith in God, and plain hard work. This dawn-to-dusk work ethic defined my upbringing. My family was my social life. My father worked extremely hard to have a successful business and we all helped where we could. He came from very modest means, and our lives were purposeful. We were your average Americans in so many important ways. Compared to the life that many have in India, we lived like royalty.

From an early age, I was given an incredible amount of responsibility. I was responsible for keeping the financial records and accounting for the money coming in. I loved it. The work was precise and results-driven. I could see a wealth of future possibilities in a spreadsheet, and I learned very early the value of a dollar. Very few young people have the opportunity to handle important financial accounting, but I became a pro. I knew my work had to be exact, or the money wouldn't add up. I began to learn and to understand the ways that money could be made and what a difference financial independence could make in the life of a family.

But I also learned that work should be balanced with light-heartedness at any age. I would see how hard my parents worked without taking enough time for themselves. It seemed like every season was a busy time for us. I would watch my mother cook, clean, work alongside my dad in the business, and do everything in her power to take care of us in the best way she knew how. She was from a generation that measured a woman's success in life by how much she gave to others. To this day, when I take an hour to get a stress-reducing massage and leave my children in my husband's very capable hands, I think of her and wonder whether she ever thought then that she deserved a massage. Now, every time she visits us, I schedule massages for her. I love watching her relax and finally taking that important time just for herself.

My success, I imagine, has been a particular point of pride for my mother. At the age of sixteen, my mother came home from school and was told she was to be married. Her dream was to become a doctor. Instead, she married my father, raised five children, and helped manage many successful family businesses. My mother embraced her destined life and cherished our family, which inspired me to follow my own dreams.

Although my mother was a model of complete selflessness, she is now sixty-four years old, and her health is not where I would like to see it. Her generation was taught to care for others. She grew up in a family where she had to take care of her mother-in-law, her several brothers-in-law, and her sisters-in-law, whom she essentially raised (my father was the eldest of eight siblings after he too, lost his eldest brother). She raised five children of her own in addition to this work. This is what a traditional Indian woman did—she got up in the morning first and she went to sleep last. Very few, if any, luxuries helped break up the work day. I believe my mother's sense of reward came from raising well-adjusted, hard-working, happy children and having a supportive and loving husband. I see my mother now and want so much for her to know how grateful I am for the sacrifices she made for us.

Sometimes the greatest lesson you learn from your parents is simply how to do things a little bit better—take time for yourself, slow down, feed your own soul, and make your own inner beauty. I think nurturing a sense of unlimited joy and peace will be even greater for my own daughter, Zoe. I feel compelled to model self-care for her so she can know herself even better than I know myself. The world has changed so much, even since I was a child. With the advent of twenty-four-hour television and the Internet, my daughter is a thousand times more at risk of being influenced and swayed by potentially negative messages regarding who she should be and how she should live her life. As a mother, I am particularly cautious about the messages that girls are bombarded with about weight, beauty, sexuality, and the complicated matter of self-worth. The best gift I can give Zoe is to live life truthfully, purposefully, consciously, and gracefully. I want our daughters, the future generation of women, to truly value, cherish, and appreciate themselves; to honor their inner and outer beauty; to have solid self-esteem; and, to have purposes that they strive toward. With each successive generation, we are slowly coming back to the essence of our own spirits and understanding that to have a grand love affair with ourselves is one of our greatest human achievements.

Although massages, spa treatments, pedicures, and naps are all nice breaks, it's critical that we begin to honor ourselves by refusing to get to the point where these temporary little delights serve to cushion the blows of life. They need to be routinely enjoyed as powerful, rejuvenating experiences that are part of a balanced wellness program that can help prevent disease and depression and ultimately empower us to improve our quality of life.

My Core Values and Beliefs

What values and beliefs do you treasure that make you

the unique and beautiful person that you are?

_____

_____

_____

_____

_____

_____

_____

_____

_____

_____

_____

_____

_____

_____

_____

_____

_____

_____

_____

_____

_____

_____

_____

_____

_____

_____

_____

_____

_____

CHAPTER 5:
THE END OF PERFECTION & THE
BEGINNING OF A NEW AGE IN SELF-CARE

"A healthy body is a guest-chamber for the soul;
a sick body is a prison"

FRANCIS BACON

For generations, women have been expected to do it all. In the 1960s and 1970s, I was a small child in a world that was dramatically changing for women. I am part of the first generation of women in this country who were taught that we can be, do, and have whatever we want in life. I wonder if young women today know that their great-grandmothers did not have the right to vote until 1920. I wonder if they realize that women could not get credit cards without the approval of their husbands or fathers until a few decades ago. And I wonder if they realize that, without incredible support, they simply *can't* do it all.

The women's movement was critical to the dignity, equality, and well-being of women in the United States and around the world. The time had come to give women the equal rights they so obviously deserved. But with that change came societal expectations that would continue to make women vulnerable socially and economically. The myth of perfection was born.

Not only could a woman work outside the home, she had to prove herself to be better than her male counterparts. At home, the responsibility of children was still primarily hers. As a wife, she still managed the affairs of the home. And, to be blunt, she had to look beautiful and to stay in a good mood while doing so to maintain marital happiness. Yes, women had equal opportunities, but they received virtually no support in grabbing and making the most of those opportunities. Women began to realize that not only is it impossible to be perfect at everything, but attempting to do so is actually quite harmful to the psyche, the spirit, and the body. No one, man or woman, can do it all.

By the 1980s, women were integrating into the workforce and beginning to routinely hold higher-level positions in government and business. But the fundamental structure of women's daily lives did *not* change. The nine-to-five work day was an invention of men. But in the modern world, where women make up the majority of workers and consumers, this schedule just doesn't make sense. Women want to mother, to work, to create, and to love. But when we're forced into an old-fashioned work paradigm, women begin to feel stretched thin and stressed out.

When I have initial consultations with my patients, I am consistently amazed at the level of work women achieve in a given day. They are breadwinners, primary caregivers, organizers, and bill payers. The stay-at-home mothers take care of their children, their elderly parents, sometimes the elderly parents of their spouses, and even work from home to make ends meet. Although men are still expected to have full-time careers, many times women are responsible for earning half the household income while still maintaining the home and raising families.

I tell my patients that striving for perfection is overrated. True perfection does not exist, and holding on to that myth can seriously damage self-esteem. I personally strive for perfect moments throughout the week—a walk with my children looking at the clouds and finding interesting things in nature; a simple dinner with my husband when we have a chance to connect, to reflect, and to fall in love all over again; time with girlfriends when we share stories, laughter, and support. Life is not perfect, and that's the way it should be.

Following is the first of nine stories told by those who say it best … my patients. They have all, in their own ways, suffered from a host of symptoms that were simply written off as "a part of life". Each of these brave women openly shares in her own words, the personal journey she took, with me by her side, to heal her broken body and spirit and successfully transform her life. This journey eventually brought her full circle to experience an enjoyable life this is meant for each of us, including you.

I commend each of these women who so courageously came to me for help and now share my mission to educate other fellow women about the importance of self-care. They have brought this message into their families, network of friends, and communities. If any of these women were having a conversation with you over a cup of coffee, she would immediately become your biggest advocate and encourage you on your own journey to Health, Happiness, and Harmony.

Cindy's Story

When I was growing up, I worshipped the sun. I loved being outside under the open sky, soaking up rays that would make my skin look healthy, young, and vibrant. My friends and I didn't know about the powerful reality of prolonged sun exposure and the sun damage that followed. And honestly, even if we had, we were young, and we just wanted to have fun and to look beautiful.

We were a family of women who liked to present ourselves well. Growing up, my mother made sure that she always looked her best. In the '40s, '50s, and '60s, I think women generally made more of an effort to look a certain way in order to be presentable. Now my mom is eighty-five years old, but what I learned from her is that when you take care of yourself, it makes you feel better. Professionally, I am also representing the interests of a large company, so I have a responsibility to look nice and to exude a positive personality. That's what people gravitate toward, and I have to cultivate that. People always used to tell me that I have it "all together." I was happy that I gave a good first impression.

But as I got older, I would get ready for the day, and I would look for that alignment between how I wanted to look and how I wanted to feel. Increasingly, I felt like I wasn't looking or feeling my best anymore. Something just wasn't right.

I began really seeing the long-term effects of sun damage, and I became concerned. I noticed that my skin looked as though it were aging prematurely. I had dark spots and wrinkles that made me feel a little self-conscious. This was troubling to me. I had always cared about the way I looked, but this was beyond my control. Internally, I was also feeling anxious and edgy for no reason—and then there were the hot flashes. I felt incapable of being in the world in the way I was used to.

So one day, I decided to do something about it—I went to visit Dr. Shel, at the recommendation of one of my girlfriends. I didn't know what to expect, and I certainly did not want to get my hopes up.

I was very honest with her about my concerns and what I was looking for. I wanted to feel beautiful again. As I was describing what I wanted, she tenderly touched my hand, and I could immediately feel her compassion. It was so reassuring, and I was touched. Here I was wearing shorts, no make-up, and looking a little sad. She had no idea that I was a successful community relations manager at a major corporation. But I was treated with dignity and concern.

We discussed my sun damage and rosacea. I knew that after time, my appearance would start to change and to improve. It was an incredible feeling to know that I could be in control of aspects of myself that I thought could never be changed. It was very liberating.

So I started my transformation externally. I thought to myself, "I have everything else under control perfectly. All I need is my face to return to a youthful glow." But I was wrong. The more I began to take stock of my well-being, the more I realized that I needed to work on my beauty from the inside out. I had maintained such a perfect façade for so long, I had not paid attention to the inner side of my health, which also needed much attention.

I was really struck by the energy level around me as I wondered if I could feel that positive, vibrant, and optimistic again. I tried so hard in my life to cultivate and to live positively. But when hormones are out of balance, as mine were, it's virtually impossible to access that side of you. After testing and discussion, I started bio-identical hormones. I immediately began to see improvements in the reduction of my hot flashes. Dr. Shel saved the day for me on that one.

For the first time in my life, I realized how important and possible it was to feel good both inside and out. I think perfection is about this need to do everything very, very well—including how you present yourself to the world. But as I began to feel better, I knew that how I felt about myself was even more important.

This was a difficult process, but I felt extremely supported know-ing that someone was there to catch me. I was on an emotional tra-peze, and Dr. Shel was my safety net. I know a lot of women feel crazy and misunderstood while their hormones are out of balance. It was such a relief to know that I'm not crazy and I don't have to just live with these hot flashes and other debilitating symptoms for the rest of my life. I actually could get rid of the anxiety I was feeling.

I finally began to understand that there was a certain type of anxiousness that came before the hot flash. I would be thinking, "What do I have to be nervous about?" Then all of a sudden, it would happen. It was scary and confusing. I truly didn't under-stand what was happening to my body. This confusion also began to affect my relationships. For no reason, my mood would suddenly change, and the claws would come out. It was damaging my rela-tionship with my husband, because when you're going through these changes, you tend to take it out on the people who are closest and dearest to you. But once I began the bio-identical hormone therapy, I started to come to my senses again and realized that I wasn't the only "mean" woman out there struggling with these symptoms. Up to that point, my body was a mystery to me. I just lived my life and tried to be great at everything I did.

The other part of this journey that I didn't expect—in addition to just having a brand-new set of information about what my body was doing and how to handle it—was a newfound knowledge of how medicine works. In traditional medicine, you feel like a number or a case file. I was a set of symptoms to be managed or cured. But in the world of integrative medicine, the doctor has to understand what is going on in my life, what my concerns are, and other personal details that can give clues about how to manage my health. It was a totally different experience. I was a real person.

After a brief time, my skin and my mood changed dramatically. I know this, because I have never received so many compliments about the way I look. It was beyond my expectations. I knew I wanted to look and to feel good again—I wanted to get back to who I really was. But I had no idea how successful the transformation would be. I feel great, and I think that shows throughout my whole body—how I carry myself, how often I smile, and just how I am with people. I think my energy level and enthusiasm for life has returned, and that makes me feel good on so many levels.

My transformation really motivates me to help other women reclaim their lives. I work at a large company, and I remember one co-worker of mine who was really going through a rough time in her marriage. I could see the physical toll it was taking on her, and I got very worried. I think some women might judge other women and say, "Oh, her hair looks terrible," or, "She's gained some weight," or, "She doesn't care about how she looks anymore." Now that I know what I know about the mind, body, and spirit connection, I have so much compassion and empathy for women who are experiencing a hiccup in their lives. I've been through that, and I came out of it much stronger and much healthier.

I took what I learned from my journey with my doctor and applied it to the relationships with women in my own life. That is how women can change the world—instead of judging one another, we can simply reach out and be a support for those among us who are going through a challenging time.

Healing is collaboration between doctors and patients, husbands and wives, friends and neighbors. Healing can happen through the positive relationships between people. As my physician, Dr. Shel provided a space for healing that was profoundly physical. But it went beyond my body—it became healing for my mind and soul, too. This collaboration has made me want to take better care of myself from now on. What an amazing gift.

One of the most rewarding aspects of my work is seeing women transform their lives before my eyes. We've all seen dramatic "before" and "after" photos highlighting incredible weight loss, youthful skin, or a new makeover. But the transformations I see are not just physical. Patients come to me with the desire to embark on re-gaining "perfection" as they experienced it at some point in their life. Generally this point in their life was when they were in their prime. They looked amazing, cherished themselves, had less stress, and were truly happy. Somewhere along the way, if we're not careful, we can lose touch with that person and these are the women I tend to every day. They often feel like they don't know where to start on their journey and it is my mission to guide them to take one step at a time and eventually we, together, will take care of both their outer beauty and inner well being, These two aspects of women directly relate to each other. Often times, I witness a complete transformation in my patients when a small positive change is made, be it with outer appearance, balanced health, or spiritual growth. Taking control of just one small part of yourself, or of your life can trigger the desire to do the same in all aspects of mind, body, spirit balancing.

Once this is achieved, the sense of peace and joy in my patients clearly emanates from the inside out. So many of my patients almost gave in to lives filled with stress, depression, and physical discomfort. Their external selves did not reflect their internal beauty. But after they received their respective treatments, they did not look back. I have seen a new generation of self-care advocates emerge, and that is amazing to me.

For many women, the idea of committing to self-care to live happier, more balanced lives is somewhat of a revolution. Taking time to meditate, to rest, to enjoy life, and to simplify requires such a different mentality than what most of us are used to. But the benefits can be profound. Imagine a world where people truly decide upon and live their own values without any outside influence. They have time to prepare nourishing food, to enjoy nature, and to connect regularly with loved ones. They have the mental and emotional strength to tackle challenges in healthy ways, and their lives are abundant with creativity and opportunity. Imagine a time in your own life when your body is in balance, providing you with the chance to explore your inner life, to have fun, and to reconnect with your spiritual source.

As women, I think we must perform important acts of self-love. In my opinion, our bodies are divine gifts; precise instruments that are intricately connected and help define who we really are. We have our human selves (our bodies and minds) and our spiritual selves (our hearts and souls). It is our mandate as we live our lives to work toward integrating these two halves to fully embrace the human experience. We came into these bodies to learn how to be human, to make choices, to heal past wounds, and to move into a divine knowing that comes when we pay attention to how we treat ourselves and others.

Now more than ever, we are becoming a global family. The influence of other cultures can be seen on every nation on Earth. America was founded on the principles of diversity and innovation, and I feel personally heartened by the fact that practices that have been common in Eastern traditions are now becoming more widely accepted by patients here in the United States. Eastern cultures share a very basic understanding that the body, mind, and soul are profoundly connected. When ailments arise, members of the Eastern cultures immediately look toward food, environmental factors, and psychological well-being as possible causes of disease. It just makes sense.

But the interests of insurance companies and pharmaceutical companies that stand to make huge profits from sick people have infiltrated basic health-care practices in the United States. Perhaps the people who should be making huge profits are organic farmers and other industries that serve the body, mind, and soul.

This is why self-care is so important. It enables us to vote for the world we want to be in with every action and choice we make. By caring for ourselves, we make healthier choices that affect everything from how corporations operate to what types of health care are available. When we support a farmers market or a health food store, a yoga studio instead of a fast-food restaurant, we are voting for a better world for ourselves and our children. When we maintain a healthy work/life balance, we are telling our colleagues that families are important. When we travel and hike through our majestic state parks, we are telling our government that protecting pristine land should be a national priority.

Yes, we have entered a new age in self-care. We are slowly beginning to see attitudes shift toward the understanding that life is to be lived, not endured. We are in the midst of a revolution that encourages people to think for themselves, to express their needs, and to become their own advocates. We now have clinical proof that living a purposeful, peaceful existence, with a sense of attaining balance as a whole person is not only good for the heart and soul but essential for physical health. Self-care is the fuel that powers our well-being and can give us the ride of our lives!

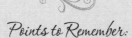

Points to Remember:

- *Perfection is in the eye of the beholder. Don't be too hard on yourself trying to attain what others have. You are a beautiful and unique woman who is perfect at all stages in her life.*

- *When trying to accomplish your goals of being the "ideal you" make sure to address what is most important to you and work from there. You can incorporate aspects of your outer physical body, your inner body, emotional well-being, and state of happiness*

- *The most important element of perfecting yourself is accepting you and expressing self-love.*

My View of Perfection

What is your view of perfection as it pertains

to you and your " ideal" self

PART TWO:

Journeys to Health

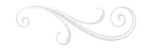

" It's never too late to become the person
you have always wanted to be"

ANNE SWEENEY

CHAPTER 6:
THE EIGHT MOST COMMON
COMPLAINTS WOMEN HAVE

"Life is not merely to be alive, but to be well"

MARCUS VALERIUS MARTIAL

After being in practice for several years, I began to see trends in the complaints and symptoms my patients were sharing with me. I couldn't ignore the fact that the vast majority of women in my care complained of these eight common symptoms (in no particular order):

1. Fatigue

2. Weight gain

3. Low sex drive

4. Hair loss

5. Skin problems

6. Mood swings

7. Depression

8. Insomnia

These were symptoms typical of menopause, but they were affecting women as young as their thirties and early forties. I began conducting my own research on the causes of these symptoms, and patient case studies repeatedly indicated that serious imbalances in thyroid, progesterone, testosterone, estrogen, cortisol, and other key hormones contributed greatly to the onset of symptoms that were severely compromising the quality of women's lives. Hormones are key components in our existence and well-being. Unfortunately, like everything else in our bodies, hormone levels also begin declining as the years pass. Different people begin declining at different ages and at different rates. It is vital that physicians and patients recognize this fact.

Furthermore, it was clear that vitamin deficiencies and food sensitivities also compromise the body's ability to function optimally. But, again, traditional physicians simply do not test for these contributing factors and often come back to suffering patients with no conclusive information that can help them. I was determined to learn everything I could about the role of hormones as well as the most state-of-the-art methodologies for identifying nutritional deficiencies. I also committed to honoring the emotional and psychological well-being of my patients. Understanding their personal lives gave me a wealth of information about stressors that could explain everything from poor lifestyle choices to increased cortisol levels and stressed adrenals. I had to know what was going on with my patients from top to bottom. I found that many of my patients were experiencing very similar symptoms that may strike a chord and resonate with your own experiences. I share their stories to show you that you are not alone.

Jan's Story

I found myself constantly looking in the mirror and saying, "Is there something wrong with me? I just don't feel like myself." At thirty-nine years old, I was a marketing executive who was overweight, depressed, and anxious all the time. My hair was falling out in clumps, and I had gained sixty pounds in a little more than a year. I felt chronically tired, unfocused, stressed out, and defeated by life. But here I was. People had told me throughout my life that I was beautiful, funny, intelligent, interesting, and with an amazing resume and a pretty decent sense of humor. I'll be honest—I stood out in a crowd. I was also a new mom to a three-year-old "spirited" little boy and was the breadwinner in my family. Not only was I the primary caretaker of our son, I brought home the bigger paycheck, managed the household finances, and still tried to keep my own creative passions intact. I was exhausted.

When I finally made the difficult decision to seek help, I think I had just concluded that life just gets harder after childbirth and the added responsibility, combined with a profound and constant lack of sleep, would be something I would simply have to push through for at least the next few years. Honestly, I didn't care how I looked, because I didn't feel all that sexy anyway. My priorities were really clear—earn enough money to keep the home fires burning while still being a present and loving mother.

I remembered so vividly a time in my life when I was a size four, walked five miles a day, meditated regularly, wore flirty skirts, experimented constantly with make-up, and went out dancing at least twice a week. I actually enjoyed a healthy, safe sex life and felt completely comfortable in my own skin.

During that time in my life, I could get a full night's sleep and wake up with a cup of tea and some fruit, feeling energized and excited about the day. Now, I was downing three cups of strong coffee and a bagel just to get in my car in the morning. I tried to take care of myself by working out and getting massages. But I still felt a strong resistance to even getting out of bed in the morning. I was married, but I felt hopeless in the relationship. I felt even more discouraged when I went to my primary care physician for a five-minute consult that resulted in a reprimand, "You have to lose the weight. Eat less and exercise more." I left with a prescription for Prozac and an utter sense of defeat.

The transformation was very alarming. I had taken such good care of myself during my pregnancy. As uncomfortable as it was sometimes, I was in the best shape of my life and never felt calmer, more at ease and in tune with my body. I regularly gave myself eight to ten hours of sleep each night. I abstained from alcohol (of course) and caffeine and all the recommended foods pregnant women are encouraged to avoid, including cold cuts, alfalfa sprouts, sushi, and more. I avoided processed foods or anything that included ingredients I couldn't pronounce. I walked or did some sort of physical activity every day and routinely took time to rest, to reflect, and to read. When I was diagnosed with gestational diabetes, I went off sugar completely and followed a nutritionist's diet to the letter. I ate six small meals a day and drank plenty of water. Throughout my pregnancy, I ate huge quantities of raw organic fruits and vegetables, envisioning those beautiful vitamins coursing into my son's precious, developing little brain and body. I was already a mother.

During that time I even rekindled my spiritual life and began meditating and praying. I monitored how I felt and what I was thinking. I knew that everything I experienced, both physically and emotionally, my son would feel also. My maternal instinct was so strong; I treated my body like a temple for the first time in my life. I would do anything to protect this vulnerable, sweet little life.

Then Dr. Shel asked me a really tough question: "Why did you stop honoring your body just because there wasn't a baby inside?" Of course, I teared up and said over and over, "I am just so tired. I don't feel like myself anymore." I admitted that I took such beautiful care of my body because I viewed it as protection and an expression of love for my unborn son. Her question challenged me to think about extending that same protection and love to myself. **While I may no longer be pregnant, there is a small, vulnerable little being resting inside each of us waiting to be loved and nurtured.**

So what was the culprit causing this downward spiral? After completing a thorough history and talking for a long time, Dr. Shel strongly suspected a severe hormonal and nutritional imbalance and possibly adrenal fatigue. She wanted to verify the levels and objec-

tive findings with some blood tests, a nutritional evaluation, and a saliva hormone test. This is the sort of testing that traditional physicians almost never do. Most physicians are trained in the medical process of cause, effect, and solution—A, then B, then C. There is no time and really no motivation to dive deep into the holistic cause of a patient's complaints. Most doctors are trained to identify the illness and to prescribe treatment to alleviate symptoms—that's it.

We talked a lot about what was going on with me, and I began to understand that my exhaustion, pain, confusion, and even deep sorrow were part of a much larger physiological and emotional picture. After the tests came back, I began a protocol of natural progesterone, natural thyroid, and natural vitamin and mineral supplements along with a healthy eating program and moderate exercise. Within three weeks, I was sleeping normally, and cravings had practically vanished. I could feel the energy race back into my cells, and a feeling of clarity and hope began to take the place of confusion and depression. Within a month, I was off Prozac for good. I began the hard work of reconciling an extremely damaged relationship with my husband. That will take time. But the good news is that the focus is back, the weight is slowly coming off, and my skin has never looked better. More than anything, I feel proud knowing that I have the strength to be the mother that I want to be and that my son deserves.

Being a Board Certified Ob/Gyn, and practicing for over a decade, I witnessed very similar situations with my postpartum patients countless times every week. I took care of women who prided themselves on cherishing and honoring their bodies and spirits while they were pregnant; however, once they delivered their babies, the desire to be unconditionally true to themselves quickly faded. I routinely heard the same symptoms. Unfortunately, being a traditional physician at the time, I ended up writing many prescriptions for anti-depressants (because I did not know any better) to help my patients simply get out of bed each day to help cope with their depression. I now understand that these women were not at all depressed, their hormones were imbalanced. I wish I knew then what I know now ... I would've been able to REALLY help those beautiful women get their lives back on track. I do often wonder about those patients of mine and hope that one day, they will find me again and get their lives and hormones balanced if they haven't already done so.

It is very common to have your maternal instinct kick in shortly after becoming pregnant, which leads to a great deal of self-care to help protect your unborn baby. This can result in women feeling the best they ever have in their lives while they are pregnant. Once you have given birth, the maternal instinct becomes even stronger and the primary focus is on the newborn; no longer on you and your body. The important point we often forget is that we all have to be good examples for our children. We need to do so by honoring ourselves and taking the best care of ourselves possible so that we are better able to provide what is needed to our loved ones. This, in turn, will set an example for them to follow that they will want to emulate. Isn't that what we want for our loved ones...for them to make their health and well-being a priority each and every day? It is up to each of us to teach our future generations how to care for themselves so they can give whole heartedly to others.

It is never too early or too late to begin caring for and loving yourself once again. You may feel alone, scared, and confused about the onset of life-changing symptoms that are completely unexplainable and new to you. You don't have to resort to simply accepting them and holding them inside. This can ultimately result in the manifestation of what feels like a downward spiral affecting the relationships within your marriage, friendships, family, and—most importantly—your close and loving relationship with yourself. Believe that you are not alone, and seek the guidance of an integrative doctor to help you reclaim what is rightfully yours—your life.

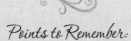

Points to Remember:

- *Through proper diagnosis, treatment, and follow-through, ancient beliefs and ways of thinking can give way to healing of the body, mind, and spirit.*

- *The need for chemical antidepressants may be reduced or eliminated entirely if you commit to a self-care regimen that empowers you to take care of yourself.*

- *Sexual dysfunction may be an indicator of larger imbalances in the body. Take your sexual health seriously to improve your overall health as well as the quality and success of your relationship with your partner.*

My Symptoms and Concerns

What symptoms do you want to
alleviate to live a healthy and happy life?

_____
_____
_____
_____
_____
_____
_____
_____
_____
_____
_____
_____
_____
_____
_____
_____
_____
_____
_____
_____
_____
_____
_____
_____
_____
_____
_____

CHAPTER 7:
THE HORMONE-REPLACEMENT MIRACLE

"A woman's health is her capital"

HARRIET BEECHER STOWE

*S*ome elements of women's health cannot be resolved simply with diet and exercise, no matter how disciplined we are. As we age, our bodies rapidly change. Think of how quickly a baby turns into a toddler, and how quickly a toddler evolves into a middle-school student. We can see the dramatic physical changes in children. We observe impressive changes in their heights and weights during their annual well-child exams. But for adults, most aging happens internally and cannot be seen except for the requisite and subtle aging of our skin, hair, posture, and stamina. It is certainly not as dramatic as shooting up four inches over summer break.

What most people don't realize is that since human beings began to wander the Earth, the typical life span was around fifty years. That's right—for most of human existence, fifty was considered a ripe old age. Biologically, our organs are still aging according to this schedule. Production of all the beneficial hormones that our organs have generated in our lifetimes—the ones that help us maintain a healthy weight; prevent mood swings, depression, and fatigue; and help us feel balanced and energetic—begins to slow down exponentially as we approach fifty. In our forties, our organs begin to say, "It's time for us to wind down now." The problem with this scenario is that humans are now living to be one hundred years old. Some studies indicate that people currently in their twenties may even live as long as one hundred twenty years–more than seventy years past the point when hormones are naturally functioning at their optimal levels. This data has huge implications for how we, as a society, will be able to take care of ourselves in our golden years. We may be living longer, but the quality of our lives is severely compromised by the fact that extended years may not be optimal in terms of functionality for our bodies.

First, let's identify the primary hormones in our bodies. The hormones that are vital to a woman's body include the sex hormones: estrogen, progesterone, and testosterone; the thyroid hormones: Triiodothyronine (T3) and Thyroxine (T4); and the adrenal hormones: DHEA-S and cortisol. They are most commonly out of balance in women due to their natural decrease in production, stress, psychological state of mind, and nutritional status. The definition of hormones, according to the *Merriam-Webster Medical Dictionary*, is "a product of living cells that circulates in body fluids (as blood) or sap and produces a specific, often stimulatory, effect on the activity of cells, usually remote from its point of origin; also called *internal secretion*."

Androgen: A steroid hormone, such as testosterone is produced primarily in the testes in men and ovaries in women. Androgen is also produced secondarily in the adrenal glands. It controls the maintenance of masculine characteristics, such as muscle and bone strength. Men produce more androgen than women, but it is necessary for both sexes to produce adequate amounts to maintain hormonal balance and physical strength in their bodies. It is also called androgenic hormones.

Testosterone: This is a steroid hormone from the androgen group that is primarily secreted in the testes of males and the ovaries of females. It is an anabolic steroid that is responsible for the development of testes, bone mass, muscle mass, and facial and body hair, and its presence is imperative to ensure a state of health and well-being in men and women. Increasing testosterone levels can be beneficial to women, because it can help increase libido and muscle mass while assisting with the treatment and prevention of depression and osteoporosis. In women, testosterone-replacement therapy is typically used in conjunction with estrogen and/or progesterone treatment. To ensure successful treatment, it is necessary to establish a baseline, to treat with bio-identical testosterone in customized doses, and to retest on an annual basis at a minimum. I do not recommend oral testosterone treatment. My method of choice is either cream or sublingual for women, and cream, sublingual, or weekly intramuscular injections for men.

Cortisol: Also known as "hydrocortisone," cortisol is a steroid hormone or glucocorticoid produced by the adrenal gland. It is released in response to physical and psychological stress as well as low levels of blood glucocorticoids. Its primary functions are to increase blood sugar through gluconeogenesis, to support the immune system, and to aid in metabolizing fat, protein, and carbohydrate. It also decreases bone formation. When we experience periods of stress, our bodies excrete cortisol to help us work through whatever the stressful situation may be. The short-term results may not be noticeable, but in the long run too much stress can lead to adrenal fatigue, which makes a perfect setting for increased inflammation in our bodies (whether joints, gastrointestinal, pelvic, or other areas) and lowered immunity, which creates numerous disease states.

Noticeable symptoms, such as weight gain, irritability, foggy thinking, chronic fatigue, and sleep disturbance, are common in people who have adrenal fatigue. Many people have misconceptions about the benefits of cortisol, because it is associated with stress. But it is an extremely valuable hormone on which nearly every bodily function relies on to reduce inflammation throughout the body, retain the ability to fight viruses and infections, improve recovery time, and maintain complete systemic immunity.

Adrenal fatigue can quickly affect hormone levels; you should have your cortisol checked along with all your sex hormones prior to any hormone replacement to ensure that your cortisol levels do not need to be corrected as well. Lifestyle modification can reverse dangerous cortisol levels dramatically, so find time to partake in stress-relieving activities, such as exercising, yoga, meditation, reading, warm baths, massages, and whatever else relaxes you. My adrenal fatigue protocol for patients includes:

- Sleep seven to eight hours every night
- Eat small, frequent meals five to six times per day
- Exercise at least three to four times per week, including cardio and strength training
- Give yourself one hour of "me time" per day, which can include any of the previously mentioned stress-relieving activities
- Take adrenal-support supplements, such as biotin, zinc, vitamin B complex, and adrenal extracts.
- Balance your hormones and nutrients
- Enjoy life and laugh more

Estrogen: Estrogen is the primary sex hormone in females. It helps promote the development of female secondary sexual characteristics, such as breasts, hips, and a wider pelvic region. Estrogen is also involved in the thickening of the endometrium and other aspects of regulating the menstrual cycle as well as preparing the body for pregnancy. It is produced in the ovaries and gradually begins to decline as a woman approaches menopause. Symptoms of estrogen imbalance can include depression, vaginal dryness, brain fog, memory loss, cognitive dysfunctions, hot flashes, night sweats, decreased bone density, fatigue, and irritability. Additional symptoms that are visible can include skin laxity, poor skin tone, dry skin, weight gain, and decreased muscle mass.

Although estrogen is present in both men and women, it is present at significantly higher levels in women of reproductive age. Numerous types of estrogen-replacement therapies are available. I would recommend that you supplement your estrogen with bio-identical estrogen, as it is derived from natural sources and is biologically identical to what your body produces; your body also has receptors for it. It is important to do your research regarding complete hormone balancing, because many women who have estrogen imbalances also have other hormone imbalances. Estrogen should not be used without progesterone, even if you've had a hysterectomy. It is very crucial to balance these two sex hormones. Be your own advocate by doing research pertaining to your symptoms and seek opinions from physicians you trust prior to treating estrogen imbalances.

Progesterone: This hormone, which is produced in the ovaries and placenta from pregnenolone, is a steroid hormone involved in the female menstrual cycle, pregnancy (supports *gestation*), and embryogenesis. Progesterone belongs to a class of hormones called "progestogens" and is the primary naturally occurring human progestogen. The main purpose of progesterone is to prepare the body for pregnancy and provide the necessary support during pregnancy to ensure the fetus is carried to term. This, however, is not the only role that progesterone plays in our bodies.

Progesterone (natural progesterone) increases libido, protects against fibrocystic breast disease, maintains the uterine lining, hydrates and oxygenates the skin, decreases hair thinning, acts as a natural diuretic, helps eliminate depression, increases a sense of well-being, encourages fat burning and the use of stored energy, and is a precursor to other important stress and sex hormones. Progesterone can also counteract symptoms in estrogen-dominant women by restoring a state of hormonal balance, happiness, and clarity as well as promoting excellent sleep. The majority of my pre- and peri-menopausal patients receive bio-identical progesterone therapy as part of their hormone treatment to regulate their periods and to help with issues concerning moods, depression, weight gain, and sleep. My menopausal patients are usually on a combination of bio-identical estrogen and progesterone (and sometimes testosterone, DHEA-S, and more) to reduce all the menopausal symptoms mentioned earlier. For a lot of women, their hormones are their life line.

Thyroid: This is one of the largest endocrine glands in the body and is not to be confused with the "parathyroid glands," which is an entirely different set of glands. The thyroid gland is found in the neck, just below the thyroid cartilage that is also known as the "Adam's Apple." The thyroid controls how quickly the body uses energy, makes proteins, and reacts to other hormones.

The thyroid gland produces thyroid hormones, principally triiodothyronine (T_3) and thyroxine (T_4). These hormones regulate the rate of metabolism and affect the growth and rate of function of many other systems in the body. Typical symptoms related to thyroid disorder include unusual changes in weight, cold body temperature, swelling in the face, dry and/or brittle hair and nails, and moodiness. Countless people suffer from these and many other symptoms, and I have found that they often are not being properly diagnosed with the thyroid conditions that they have. It is essential to your health to have a physician/health-care provider who will listen to your symptoms and take them into as much consideration as your lab results, thus assisting you in achieving optimal health.

In my practice, I have found that the vast majority of my patients experienced very similar symptoms, so I developed a symptoms checklist. When most of my patients first view this list, recognition, relief, and excitement come over them as they realize they are not the only ones with these symptoms. In other words, there are hundreds of women you may know who are experiencing the same myriad of debilitating symptoms. The question is: When will all these women take control of their lives?

Hormone Checklist

As an exercise to help you determine what hormonal imbalances you may have based on symptoms alone, check the symptoms that apply to you. If you check more than 5 symptoms listed, you should seek the care of an Integrative Physician who can conduct the appropriate testing to determine your hormonal imbalances and correct them with bio-identical replacement options.

Feel free to visit my practice website for more in-depth symptom questionnaires that are very specific to commonly overlooked diagnoses.

www.drshel.com

Estrogen Imbalance (Dominance or Deficiency)

___Hot Flashes	___Depression	___Fibrocystic Breasts
___Night Sweats	___Sleep Disturbance	___Tender Breasts
___Vaginal Dryness	___Heart Palpitation	___Uterine Fibroids
___Foggy Thinking	___Bone Loss	___Water Retention
___Memory Lapses	___Dry Skin/Hair	___Weight Gain (Hips)
___Incontinence	___Headaches	___Nervousness
___Tearfulness	___Mood Swings (PMS)	___Bleeding Changes
___Irritability	___Breast Cancer	___Cold Body Temp

Progesterone Imbalance

___*Candida* Infections	___Fluid Retention	___Sleep Disturbance
___Fibrocystic Breasts	___Arthritis	___Break-thru Bleeding
___Hair Loss	___Endometriosis	___Weight Gain
___Anxiety	___Hyper Stress	___Heavy Periods
___Headaches	___Water Retention	___PMS
___Depression	___Mood Swings	___Cramps
___Irritability	___Insomnia	___Irregular Cycles

Androgen Imbalance

___Low Libido	___Depression	___Memory Lapses
___ Oily Skin	___Ovarian Cysts	___Excessive Body Hair
___Vaginal Dryness	___Sleep Disturbance	___Increased Acne
___Fatigue	___Thinning Pubic Hair	___Hair Loss (Scalp)
___Heart Palpitations	___Incontinence	___Thinning Skin
___Bone Loss	___Elevated Triglycerides	___Fibromyalgia
___Aches/Pains/ Arthritis	___Nervousness/ Irritability	___Decreased Muscle Mass
___Excessive Facial Hair		

Cortisol Imbalance		
___Cold Body Temp	___Sleep Disturbance	___Anxiety
___Memory Lapse	___Irritability	___Bone Loss
___Allergies	___Arthritis	___Headaches
___Acne	___Heart Palpitations	___Fatigue
___Stress	___Aches/Pains	___Weight Gain/Loss
___Nervousness	___Muscle Mass Loss	___Sugar Cravings
___Thinning Skin	___Low Libido	___Hair Loss
___Elevated Triglycerides	___Chemical Sensitivity	
Thyroid Imbalance		
___Cold Hands & Feet	___Low Blood Pressure	___Hair Loss
___Slow Pulse Rate	___Mood Changes	___Forgetfulness
___Cold Body Temp.	___Decreased Sweating	___Memory Lapse
___Weight Gain/ Loss	___Difficulty Concentrating	___Fatigue or Exhaustion
___Sadness or Depression	___Swelling/Puffy Eyes/Face	___Inability to Lose Weight

Once you know your symptoms, a thorough review of your history and hormone testing are the first steps to regaining your wellness and sense of self. Testing can be done with either saliva or blood tests. However, insurance companies typically do not want to pay for these tests. This stonewalling becomes the first harsh reality when patients enter the world of integrative medicine— the insurance and pharmaceutical industries, for all intents and purposes, direct and drive the traditional medical community.

Even the "desired levels" of hormones have been established by the traditional medical community. But some laboratories, such as ZRT Laboratories, Neuroscience,

Diagnos- Tech, and others, have created a more accurate range for hormone levels when tested with saliva and bloodspot.

The bottom line is that women are systemically being told that their hormone levels "are within range." But who created that range? The truth is: these standard ranges that we have all become accustomed to are actually very large – spanning from one end of the spectrum to the other. More importantly, the rise of integrative medicine and treating within a very small range has proven that these large, vast ranges do not support optimal health and are quite possibly going to be a thing of the past. Why are so many women's lives being transformed and healed as a result of a more accurate hormone diagnosis using integrative standards and methodologies? How is it that new standards are being set to respond to a mass need for hormonal health that actually makes women healthier, happier, and more balanced?

The answer lies in the integrative medical community's unwavering commitment to treat women not as a group but as whole individuals with individual chemical and hormonal structures that require personal attention and response. A battle has developed between compassion and healing for the individual and mass production for groups of consumers. At every stage in human history up to this point—with the sole exception of battlefield medics—doctors had been trained to meet the needs of the unique individual. Now people are being treated based on mass ranges, mass diagnoses, and mass prescription recommendations. The battle for women's health is fully underway.

In the field of hormone-replacement therapy, the market currently offers two distinct kinds of hormones: synthetic and natural (also referred to as "bio-identical" hormones). Synthetic hormones are artificially formulated with chemical structures that can work similarly to natural hormones, but in most cases their compositions vary significantly. Natural hormones are derived from plants and are chemically the same as your body's intrinsic hormones. By using plant-based natural hormones, you are extending the function of hormones that occur naturally in your own body, because the compound of these hormones is exactly like the hormones you produce. By their very nature, bio-identical hormones aid in producing normal levels in your body's hormone profile.

In the world of bio-identical or compounded hormones, patients are given the unique opportunity to receive customized hormones. This is a revolutionary treatment concept. Patients are no longer at the mercy of prescriptions where dosage levels are equivalent to non-customized care. In the case of bio-identical hormone-replacement treatment, each patient receives a different compound depending on where her individual deficiencies are found. For example, if estradiol is sold by Company A, it might come in .05, .1, and .2 doses. But what if the patient needs a .75 dose or a 2.75 dose? How does this patient get what she really needs rather than what is simply "close enough"? How do we avoid compromising the beneficial results?

The mode of delivery for certain hormones is also extremely critical. For estrogen and testosterone specifically, it's important that you not take those hormones orally; because they can impact your liver function, which, in turn, can increase your triglyceride levels. Yet when pharmaceutical companies recommend hormones, they are usually offered in their oral form –the current standard. Again, this is problematic, because delivery methods from pharmaceutical companies are uniform, not customized.

What's the better option? Compounded hormones– sometimes in the form of creams instead of oral forms–can be much more customized. One patient may receive a cream with a number of different recommended hormones customized specifically for her, such as specific levels of estradiol, estriol, progesterone, testosterone, and DHEA.

Women are not accustomed to believing that hormones can be effective if they are applied topically. We've been conditioned to believe that medicine must be taken orally. But the fact of the matter is that what goes *on* your body goes *in* your body. Your skin is your largest organ, and the ingredients in topical creams can quickly be absorbed into your tissues. This fact is also why I recommend that my patients wear mineral-based make-up to keep harmful chemicals away.

Just as it is very important to find the right Integrative Physician to address your hormonal imbalance, it is equally important to use the best pharmacies that specialize in hand making your hormones specific to your needs. Special compounding pharmacies must be licensed and regulated to produce bio-identical hormones. Patients should consult with their physicians to find safe and reputable compounding pharmacies that are accredited by the Compounding Pharmacies Accreditation Board (CPAB) or the Pharmaceutical Compounding Accreditation Board (PCAB), which only use ingredients from Professional Compounding Centers of America (PCCA). Following these suggestions will ensure that your body gets the highest quality of Bio-Identical Hormones with the best absorption rate to begin alleviating symptoms and ultimately balancing your hormones.

Compounded hormones are much closer to what we produce naturally. Most integrative physicians determine appropriate dosage based on objective and subjective findings. The reality is that most traditional physicians don't even check hormone levels, because they assume that if the patient is menopausal, that woman automatically needs estrogen or progesterone in standard dosing. These doctors may have more of a "hit or miss" approach to the dosage, which is not very effective. In my practice, I use bio-identical hormones that, when compounded perfectly, mimic precisely the hormones that naturally occur in the body, thus returning the feeling of optimal well-being the patients once experienced. This is what most women are searching for—to feel how we once felt in our youth.

I subscribe to the guidelines of the American College of Obstetricians & Gynecologists and practice with the philosophy of using the lowest, most effective dose of hormones while my patients are symptomatic. The only differing issue here is that most traditional doctors believe that menopausal symptoms only include hot flashes and night sweats. How about symptoms of depression, mood swings, irritability, loss of libido, weight gain, hair loss, fatigue, and so on? Are we just expected to live with those? Or do we stop the hormones and begin taking antidepressants to mask those symptoms and subsequently gain even more weight? This is where my philosophy differs. I believe the symptoms listed above are generally related to hormonal imbalance and are real issues during the peri- and postmenopausal years. This fact cannot be ignored. Patients ask me: "How long will I need to use the bio-identical hormones?" My answer is very simple: "How long do you want to feel good?"

This is where quality-of-life issues come into play. Sure, the media and other sources will cite many studies (many of which are not done very well, although some are better than others) that will certainly scare you or make you question whether you should be using hormones at all—synthetic or bio-identical. I spend a lot of time counseling my patients on the risks, benefits, and alternatives to using bio-identical hormones. Statistically speaking (according to studies), one in eight of us will get breast cancer. Look around you and count eight of your friends—one, if not more, of you will unfortunately suffer from this disease. Scary, isn't it? What can you do to decrease your chances? So much of living a healthy life is common sense and is widely known already: eat a healthy diet, exercise, avoid harmful substances, and take the correct vitamins, minerals, and antioxidants.

Do you miserably live in fear of getting cancer? Do you assume that not using bio-identical hormones will prevent it? Unfortunately, this is not the case. Many factors influence getting any type of cancer. Women want to be well today and feel great. Most women are not concerned about a miniscule, increase in their chances of getting cancer. Most of my patients have read all the papers, articles, and blogs before entering my office. They have chosen quality of life, freedom, optimal health, balance, harmony, and womanhood. They want their old selves back!

Felicia's Story

I had spent my entire adult life creating a home and family that was beautiful, stable, and very close-knit. I was so proud of how connected we all were and equally proud of my marriage—we're high-school sweethearts. I met Dan when I was fifteen years old and in the tenth grade. After high school, we got married and eventually moved with my husband's company when I was seven months' pregnant with my daughter. I was nineteen. Except for my husband, I was alone and pregnant, but I considered myself very strong. I was creating traditions all by myself as a young mother, but I loved it. I had my twenty-first birthday when I was seven months' pregnant with my son, Brian. Then, I had another beautiful daughter. All in all, I felt very content with the direction of my life.

After the children were grown and out of the house, life changed quite a bit. For my entire adult life, I had given and given and given. So now I was thrust into the harsh reality of an empty nest. I had no idea how to feel or what to do.

People ask me sometimes why I dedicated my life to my family the way I did. The bottom line is that it has always been just the five of us. We have no extended family nearby, so our children didn't under-stand the concept of aunts, uncles, grandparents, and cousins. As a result, we were very close-knit, because that's all we had. We would have occasional visits to family out of state, or they would some-times come to visit. But overall, extended-family interactions were not part of our regular family life. And because of that, I was really the nucleus of the family.

You see, my family is extremely perceptive, and we're all very much tuned in to each other. I am certain that they believe if Mom's not happy, then no one is happy. My job as a mom and a wife was to keep the household going in the right direction, so however I felt at any given moment always really influenced the general mood of the house.

I think it's important to understand how powerful that role really is. My husband is an executive, and he does very well for us. But as my personality began to change, he started to feel that his hard work was pointless, because it didn't seem like anyone in our family was really happy. It was distressing. He began to feel unappreciated and under terrible stress and pressure. In my experience, men don't have an emotional network like women naturally do. They don't seek emo-tional support from each other. They receive that support from their wives, more often than not. So when I began to check out emotionally, I believe my husband was really lost. This had never happened before, and I was confused about why my moods were becoming so extreme.

As a result, his pain and frustration would occasionally come out after one cocktail too many. And one night, everything came to a head. In passing, my son mentioned to me that my husband had said that we were probably going to get a divorce. My initial reaction surprised me—I was furious.

In a strange way, I was proud of myself for being so angry. It meant that I still had some strength inside that I could draw from during this challenging time. Though I didn't really feel like myself, I knew right then and there that I had to go in search of myself. The troubles with my husband had triggered something very important in my life. I just felt crazy, scared, and out of control. But on some level, I knew that it wasn't just the situation at hand. I knew that something out of the ordinary was happening to me on a physical level that made me scramble to understand why I felt so lethargic, apathetic, and miserable. I think that was the first time I really began to understand the powerful connection between the mind and the body.

Overall, I just felt like I was "losing it." One day, I tuned in to a TV show where Dr. Shel was being interviewed. She spoke about hormonal imbalances, low energy, sleep disorders, depression, and so many other conditions that I immediately identified with. She talked about how women constantly take care of others while neglecting themselves. I thought, "This is me! I have to meet her. I need help." I called my girlfriend and asked if she'd like to go with me, and she said, "Yes." I was still so mad, but I made the decision that I was going to go on this journey for myself, and for no one else. I'm taking control, I'm looking after me. I didn't want to be one of those people who wakes up one day and realizes that you've devoted all your good years to someone and that person gets to decide your fate. I don't think so.

I wanted to find out about my hormones first. If that checked out fine, then what would I do? I really didn't want to take antidepressants, and I didn't want to depend on the "medication bandage," so to speak. I really wanted to say, "This isn't normal. I'm not feeling right. I'm not myself—what's going on?" It was a complete sense of confusion and concern that initially motivated me.

Even though I was physically active, the truth was that I was not regularly exercising. I just wasn't focused, in part because I had resigned myself to being a certain weight, almost as though my body had decided to be in the mid-180s and size twelve or size fourteen. I consider myself forever a size twelve to fourteen. I was an attractive lady, so I basically felt resigned to it. But emotionally, I had gotten to the point that I wasn't getting out of bed, and I just didn't care anymore.

I wasn't sleeping, and I felt like my life was spinning out of control and I wanted off. I couldn't deal with my life as it was and simply told myself, "I'm done." I was probably in a depressive state, which I knew was very dangerous. But I did feel that enough of "me" was still present that I was aware that I had severe hormonal imbalances or I just needed to get on antidepressants. But I was reluctant to go the latter route. I had to do something, because on the one hand I wasn't sleeping. On the other hand, I couldn't get out of bed. I guess I was avoiding life. When daylight would come, I couldn't even get out of bed to face the day.

So when I went to seek help from Dr. Shel, I was desperate. I didn't really know what to expect. She talked about the hormone-replacement therapy, and it hit me that I might be suffering from some hormonal issues that were totally out of my control. I wasn't handling problems well, and everything seemed so magnified, so that every little thing just felt huge. Every task was just too much.

When I finally had my consult with her, I started to cry, because, after listening to me carefully and evaluating me, everything she said started to make sense. It seemed so logical that if your adrenal glands are stressed, you're not going to handle things as easily as you normally would. She went on to explain that it is perfectly natural that if you are making too much cortisol and too little thyroid, you won't lose weight. Also, if you are estrogen dominant and progesterone deficient, you are susceptible to mood swings and depression. I committed to getting hormonally and nutritionally balanced. I began to embrace a healthy lifestyle and cherish myself. I finally exhaled and thought, "I can do this."

Once I felt more balanced, I started diving into the reality of my weight situation. I was talking about feeling complacent and okay *with where I was with my weight. But after my test results came back, I was placed on progesterone cream, thyroid medication, and several natural supplements, including one for sleep. I immediately began sleeping better, and I couldn't believe how wonderful I felt. I felt so proud that I was going through this process for myself. I even began the journey right before the holidays, because I wanted this to be about a real commitment to myself, without excuses. And the holidays were wonderful. I still cooked and baked, but I put my health and well-being on the top of my priority list, and it stayed that way. I could have made all the excuses in the world, and I could have waited until after the holidays, but the point was that I was making this life change for myself. I took control right then and right there. It felt amazing.*

I thought I had been in control for all the years I was raising my family. But I've learned that I had lost some of my power along the way. Now, whatever happens in my life is up to me and my own choices. My husband and children have their paths and destinies, which I will always respect and support. But I have mine, too. I've never really felt like that before.

I was forty-three then, and one of my main concerns was that I wanted to be in control of what the next twenty years of my life would be like. I knew that the decisions I make right now are going to determine what the next chapter of my life would look like. My mother is morbidly obese, and she has all the health problems that go along with that. My sister is three years older than I am. I can't get her to stop smoking or to take care of herself. I wanted to break the cycle of unhealthy habits in my family.

This whole experience has been an awakening, and I feel truly empowered . . . and feeling empowered is sexy. Confidence in general is sexy. I finally feel like I am driving my own life. Now, I will never feel vulnerable to someone else's decisions again. And one of the wonderful results of my newfound health is that my husband is my greatest fan. He's so proud of how far I've come and says he admires and respects my achievements. Our marriage is better than ever. That's why I think it's important to say to women, "You're okay. It's going to be okay. Don't worry. There really is hope."

There is hope for everyone. It is my personal and professional mission to reach as many women as I can, so they know they don't have to feel hopeless. I want them to know that everything truly is going to be okay. The scariest step can be admitting that you don't feel like yourself and then convincing yourself that you can change this situation with your commitment to your health and by getting under the care of an Integrative Physician. There is a delicate balance that needs to be maintained between thyroid, cortisol, and sex hormones. If only one of these essential anti-aging components becomes out of balance, eventually the others will follow and ultimately decline. This is why I believe in testing patients for their thyroid and cortisol levels as well prior to starting any hormone treatment regimen. This allows the body to quickly begin to restore a state of health instead of continuing to compensate for the areas that would otherwise go un-treated, and eventually create more health issues.

When your hormones are compromised, some personal time to reduce stress, healthy diet modifications, and deeper self-reflection to figure out why you feel like someone else, may be helpful to some degree; however, the deeper rooted issues need to be addressed to close the loop on your health. Taking care of yourself first and foremost before all others in your life is the key to living a long healthy life. Appreciate yourself and make yourself a priority by becoming your own best friend. If your best friend or a family member were struggling, would you not provide compassion, understanding, and advice? Would you not follow up with that person's wellness until he or she were whole again? Give yourself the same consideration and love that you give to others by taking control of your wellness sooner rather than later.

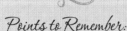

Points to Remember:

- *Once you become educated in the complex powers of hormones in your life, you can become an advocate for other women to seek out the latest information on hormone health.*

- *Believe in a course of trial and error. Be willing to adapt and be flexible with your treatment. Allow for adjustments and evaluations as you move toward health and well-being.*

- *Hundreds of new resources are available online regarding hormone health that will empower patients to become partners with their health-care practitioners. Seek them out and become a student of your own body.*

My Checklist of Symptoms

How do your symptoms impact your life?

Refer to your list of symptoms on the hormone checklist.

_____
_____
_____
_____
_____
_____
_____
_____
_____
_____
_____
_____
_____
_____
_____
_____
_____
_____
_____
_____
_____
_____
_____
_____

CHAPTER 8:
FROM PHYSICAL CHAOS TO ULTIMATE
BALANCE—ADRENAL FATIGUE

"Don't count the days, make the days count"

MUHAMMAD ALI

*A*drenal fatigue results when the adrenal glands function below the necessary level. Most commonly associated with intense or prolonged stress, it can also arise during, or after, acute infections or illnesses. As the name suggests, its main symptom is fatigue that is not relieved by sleep; however, it is not a readily identifiable entity like hypertension. You may look and act relatively normal with adrenal fatigue and may not have any obvious signs of physical illness, yet you live with an overall sense of feeling depressed, tired, and lethargic. People experiencing adrenal fatigue often have to use coffee, caffeinated beverages, and other stimulants to get going in the morning and to keep themselves up during the day.

Although it affects millions of people in the U.S. and around the world, conventional medicine does not yet recognize it as a distinct syndrome. Most physicians don't even list it in their differential diagnoses when a patient goes in with extreme, chronic fatigue. More often than not, traditional physicians have never tested their patients for this. Adrenal fatigue can wreak havoc on your life. In the more serious cases, the activity of the adrenal glands is so low that you may have difficulty getting out of bed for more than a few hours per day. With each level of reduction in adrenal function, every organ and system in your body is more profoundly affected. Changes occur in your metabolism, thyroid and hormonal balance, gastrointestinal and cardiovascular system, and even sexual function. Many other alterations take place at the biochemical and cellular levels in response to the adrenals not functioning well. Your body does its best to make up for the malfunctioning adrenal glands, but it does so at a price.

Adrenal fatigue is produced when your adrenal glands cannot sufficiently meet the demands of stress. What I have seen over the years is that adrenal fatigue occurs when your stress has taken a toll, affected your body to the point that your hormone and nutritional profiles are so out of balance that the body physically shuts down. Symptoms of adrenal fatigue include weight gain, exhaustion, insomnia, mood swings, and depression. Adrenal fatigue can present itself in symptoms that may mimic other conditions, which leaves patients confused and unfortunately, often times, misdiagnosed. In my practice, I often see very accomplished women who drive themselves to the point of their bodies shutting down.

It pains me to see women drive themselves so hard that they begin to define themselves in terms of what they do for a living. I encourage my patients to look deep within themselves to ask the simple question, "Who am I?" This so rarely ends up being about what you do. Rather, it becomes a question of whether you are living with integrity according to your most heartfelt values. High on the list of most people's priorities is "good health," yet often we take this most vital aspect of our existence for granted. All too often, it is overlooked and not given the appropriate attention it needs. Good health is not simply living free of disease, it is the prevention of disease accompanied by a well balanced life. I hope that as women walk their unique paths to well being, they begin to really treasure, appreciate, and cherish who they are. Each and every one of them is a valuable and beautiful person who deserves the best health. Most importantly, they each need to provide themselves with the opportunity and time to give this gift on a daily basis to attain and maintain their healthy state of wellness.

Cara's Story

Feeling like your body is basically shutting down is a terrible sensation. You feel like you can't move. You want to stay in bed, sleep, and just sink into the sheets and pull the covers over your head. It feels like you have the flu, but you don't. So, the complete exhaustion and fatigue is even more confusing and concerning.

It was January, and I had been to cardiologists, gastroenterologists, and psychologists to find out why I felt so tired. I was tested for sleep apnea and even underwent a series of blood and nuclear stress tests. I eagerly anticipated test results and feedback from the medical professionals I was turning to for help in hopes of receiving answers to my medical dilemma. But, over and over again, I was told that everything was fine—I just had a "little hormone or chemical imbalance." Nothing was wrong with me. This made me feel even more desperate and exhausted—I felt like I couldn't function normally in the world. It was scary and strange. I would lose two or three days at a time staying in bed, and my family was beginning to worry.

I began hearing about adrenal fatigue and bio-identical hormone therapy and finally scheduled an appointment with Dr. Shel based on my therapist's recommendation. I wanted to make sure that I let her know I was not depressed and I did not want to be on antidepressants. Psychologically, my angst was linked to the fact that I physically could not function. But it seemed as though I had the symptoms of depression, and I just needed to get to the bottom of it. I told her I felt "fuzzy-headed," and I was not able to balance my day-

to-day obligations, including taking care of my kids and running my business.

I had also experienced several major upheavals in the previous months. I lost my office during Hurricane Ike and had to temporarily relocate my business. At the age of forty-seven, my brother had quintuple bypass surgery, and my mother had a serious stroke. Dr. Shel was the first doctor to help me explore how my practical life experiences were contributing to my condition.

My assistant was very concerned, because I wasn't leading the business the way I normally did. This was completely out of character for me. I had always taken great pride in my success, and I was absolutely devoted to my business and my career. She kept imploring me to "slow down," but I didn't listen, and then everything just came to a screeching halt. My husband didn't know what to do, and my kids were walking on eggshells. They never knew if I was going to be happy or sad when I walked through the door. They didn't know whether I was going to snap at them or hug them. It was very stressful for everyone.

Once Dr. Shel evaluated me carefully and thoroughly, she recommended I begin with a Myers cocktail; this is an intravenous drip filled with high doses of vitamins and minerals to help replenish the nutrients that she clinically suspected I was lacking. She then assisted me in the detoxification process of my body. I instantly felt a burst of energy, and within a few days. I began feeling refreshed and a lot clearer.

We proceeded with checking my sex-hormones, intracellular nutrient levels with SpectraCell, my thyroid, and my adrenal hormones. It was a complete top-to-bottom evaluation. The tests concluded that I was menopausal and in adrenal fatigue; I was placed on an individualized program that consisted of bio-identical hormones, a small dose of cortisol, adrenal extracts, thyroid and customized nutritional supplementation. I was instructed to reduce my stress; to begin yoga and meditation; to get massages when possible and to take time for myself. I needed to drink more water. It was recommended for me to sleep at least 7-8 hours per night (which I rarely did), and I was placed on a moderate exercise program that included cardiovascular and resistance exercises. Finally, it was all about me. For the first time in my life, I was the most important person, and I was told by Dr. Shel, "You either commit to taking care of you or you lose you! This is entirely your choice. Only you can help yourself"

In less than two months, I was seeing a significant change. I was able to get out of bed, and I felt refreshed. I was able to start functioning better and stopped my antidepressants. I was finally taking care of myself, and my energy level picked up dramatically. I wasn't dragging, and I could really see a big difference. By September, my children still thought I was on antidepressants and anti-anxiety medications! I wasn't. My assistant saw a significant change, too. By that December, I felt like I was back to my old self. It was incredible! I was just amazed.

While I know it was hard for my daughters, who were twelve and sixteen at the time, I'm glad they had the chance to see firsthand the power of hormones and how to take control of your own health. I want them to be diligent about advocating for their own health and to not give up until they find something that works. In my case, they saw that the treatment was really changing my life for the better, and as a result, I could participate more fully in their lives. That's exactly what I wanted and what they really needed.

Finding help and getting better is such a wonderful feeling. My family is so grateful that I found somebody who could give me the help I desperately needed. I think this process has actually brought me and my family closer together.

I learned a lot from this experience. Now, I feel great. I sleep well at night, and I get up refreshed in the morning. My days are really good. I'm able to juggle, but also I'm more able to relax and to slow down when needed. It's made me realize that the most important *assets in my life are my health and my family. This experience has given me a better perspective on everything, and I now make having an appropriate work/life balance a major priority.*

We have all heard that stress reduction contributes to an improved state of health, but it goes far beyond the well known lowering of cardiac risks. Stress is directly linked to adrenal function, which can either promote health when stress is low and manageable, or it can cause failure in all systems in your body when it is not balanced with stress-reducing practices. It seems that our daily lives have become more stressful as we take on more challenges, have more to accomplish, and have less time to care for ourselves. Now, more than ever, stress reduction habits need to be established and incorporated into our lives every day to restore a healthy balance so our bodies can thrive.

Balance is the key to experiencing life as it was intended for each of us. It is hard to determine which came first: the lack of balance and excess stress leading to poor health or the decline in health that leads to the lack of balance and life-changing onset of symptoms. Regardless of which came first, all types of stress can ultimately lead to adrenal fatigue, chronic inflammation, a compromised immune system, and overall decline in health. My goal with patients is to determine what imbalances need to be corrected on a physical level, to provide the proper treatments, and then to complete the wellness loop by incorporating mental, emotional, and psychological aspects to their specific treatment plan. This goal enables my patients to be treated based upon *who they are*, what their day-to-day lives consist of, and *what their bodies physically need.* I treat each of my patients as they deserve to be treated—as a complex and multi-dimensional woman. When you make the decision to seek out the care of an integrative physician, I encourage you to find one that keeps all aspects of *you* at the heart of the goals and treatments to ensure proper attention and care.

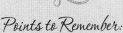

Points to Remember:

- *Do not give in to the idea that getting older means getting progressively less active and increasingly tired. More often than not, changes in hormones account for a large part of the fatigue we feel on a daily basis.*

- *Use your health pitfalls to reevaluate what is important in life. Ask yourself if working much more than simply living and enjoying life is providing you with the quality of life that you're looking for?*

- *Consider reprioritizing your responsibilities and using your cherished free time to care for yourself and spend time with loved ones.*

My Idea of Balance and Harmony.

How can you make more time for "being" rather than "doing".
What are your main priorities and why?

_____
_____
_____
_____
_____
_____
_____
_____
_____
_____
_____
_____
_____
_____
_____
_____
_____
_____
_____
_____
_____
_____
_____
_____
_____
_____

CHAPTER 9:
THE SECRETS OF VITAMINS & NATURAL SUPPLEMENTS

"To ensure good health: Eat lightly, breathe deeply, live moderately, cultivate cheerfulness, & maintain interest in life"

WILLIAM LONDEN

Generations ago, life was much simpler. Most people received a fairly adequate supply of vitamins through food, water, and sunshine. Food was less processed, so it was more easily digestible. With fewer stressors, the immune system did not have to work quite as hard to pull nutrients into the body. Today, our bodies are ravaged by internal and external factors such as: processed foods, environmental exposure to pollution, and chemicals which are found in every day simple items such as common household cleaners. The overexposure we experience on a daily basis puts an incredible strain on our ability to extract and to absorb the nutrients we need to remain in a balanced and healthy state. Combine that with busy lifestyles, and we are in nutritionally precarious positions. That's why it is so important for you to take vitamins and nutritional supplements. However, even after the commitment is made, it is difficult to determine which ones are most effective. Information about supplements can be overwhelming, and not everyone is qualified to provide correct and complete advice on which ones are best.

In my practice, once I complete a thorough evaluation along with a history of symptoms, I am better able to determine if a nutritional deficiency is likely. Often, a deficiency is evident and I recommend a nutritional assessment by SpectraCell Laboratories. This advanced test detects individual intracellular deficiencies of thirty-three different vitamins, minerals, and antioxidants, including eight B vitamins, including B12 and biotin; amino acids; calcium; vitamins D, E, A, C; selenium; CoQ10; magnesium; and other antioxidants. I then counsel the patient and customize a unique supplementation program for each individual based on their individual and unique symptoms and nutritional deficiencies.

It is also extremely important to take the correct supplements manufactured by the best companies. There is a huge difference between over-the counter supplements that you can purchase at a myriad of vitamin stores, drugstores, and organic food stores; as compared to those purchased from companies that are very seriously regulated and are held to very high standards by regulatory companies to produce supplements that actually contain the ingredients that are listed on the label, in the correct amounts, are truly absorbable by our bodies, and have minimal to no fillers and binders that have no nutritional value for our bodies. Beware of claims made by generic companies that are sold at the above mentioned vitamin retail places. The more reputable companies can only distribute their supplements via healthcare providers' offices, such as physicians, naturopathic doctors, chiropractors, etc. Do your own research and put into your bodies what you know is high quality and well-absorbed.

On countless occasions, I have seen patients who come in with a bag full of vitamins that they've been taking for years and spending hundreds of dollars on per month. When I test them for their intracellular deficiencies, they are very deficient on the very vitamins and minerals that they've been taking for a very long time. Why? This is because most of them were over the counter supplements which are not regulated and unfortunately, do not have what they claim to have in them, in the correct doses, or simply may not be absorbable in our bodies. This is precisely why I recommend medical grade supplements for my patients by a few very specific companies that I have researched, tested, and confirmed. I do not want my patients, or anybody for that matter, to waste their hard earned money on products that simply do not work. Some of my favorite nutritional supplement companies are as follows: Douglas Laboratories for most essential nutrients, minerals and antioxidants; Transformation Enzymes for most gut related issues such as probiotics, digestive enzymes and proteases; Thorne for Biotin; and a few others that you can reference on my website. www.drshel.com.

The traditional medical community continues to flounder on exploring the relationship between nutrition and disease. Instinctively, we know that we are what we eat, but the health-care system still does not place a premium on prevention and becoming nutritionally balanced to stave off serious illness.

While there are countless supplements that may be needed by the body based on individual evaluations, there is, one extremely important supplement that I recommend to all of my patients, both male and female, regardless of nutritional status. Fish oil is a supreme supplement that is beneficial for everyone regardless of their dietary intake. I only recommend high quality fish oil which is made from the oily tissue of such fish as trout, salmon, tuna, sardines, and more. This life-enhancing oil offers essential omega-3 fatty acids, such as eicosapentaenoic acid (EPA) and decosahexaenoic acid (DHA), which have specific health benefits, including fighting mental illnesses such as bipolar disorder and depression, and even reducing the risk of heart disease and heart attacks. Fish oil has the unique ability to lower a certain form of blood fat called triglycerides and to increase HDL, or what experts call "good" cholesterol. Fish oil has also been reported to prevent strokes and abnormal heart rhythms as well as to lower blood pressure and slow the hardening of arteries. Additionally, omega-3 fatty acids from fish oil can decrease inflammation throughout the body, which can result in a reduction of myriad complications, including cancer, Alzheimer's, psoriasis, and autoimmune diseases.

Fish oil also helps with minor conditions, including morning stiffness, arthritic pain, and everyday stiffness in the joints. On yet a more basic level, fish oil helps lengthen the lifespan of cells, essentially slowing the physical aging process. Other extraordinary benefits include better eyesight, increased brain function, and more restful and sound sleep. It's a natural and highly powerful addition to your daily self-care regimen but only if it is a high-quality, medical grade fish oil.

My other highly recommended supplement for women is Diindolmethane (DIM). DIM is a natural Antioxidant and Phytonutrient found in cruciferous vegetables such as broccoli, cauliflower, and brussel sprouts. It is a metabolite of Indole-3-carbinol (I3C) and is the most active plant indole (organic compound) that promotes positive estrogen metabolism. The metabolic enzymes in DIM are similar to hormone balancing enzymes naturally occurring in our bodies. It has been used for over 10 years to maintain healthy hormonal balance, and has recently been discovered to be natural alternative for breast cancer prevention. This is another "must" supplement for most of my female patients who may be dealing with either PCOS (Polycystic Ovarian Syndrome), fibroids, breast issues, irregular menses, or simply who want to be healthy and prevent issues relating to estrogen dominance as we discussed in Chapter 7.

Although everyone can benefit from many supplements, it is important to recognize the fact that we are all individuals therefore, we all absorb our nutrients differently. Additionally, over-the-counter and prescription medications can deplete our nutritional statuses, and the foods we eat are not as nutrient-packed as they were years ago. I can't stress enough the importance of nutritional-deficiency testing, such as SpectraCell micronutrient testing, to determine which vitamins and minerals you are lacking. You may be taking a handful of vitamins every day because advertising and articles tell you to take them; but you are a unique individual with a unique set of nutrients that your body may need more or less of. The benefits of a nutritionally balanced body are multi-fold. It greatly improves the quality of life while supporting and protecting it from diseases.

Lois's Story

I am a woman in my fifties with a busy life, a flourishing career, two grown daughters, and a loving husband. I am happy to say that I am also a grandmother. All seemed to be more or less well in my world. This view was supported by my spiritual life. I always considered myself a pretty conscientious person who felt in tune with both my inner and outer self. But something just didn't feel right.

In addition to being spiritual, I am also very health conscious— probably more than most. I always took vitamins regularly and always maintained some sort of exercise program. I was a firm believer in taking care of myself and being the best person I could be. But suddenly it hit me—I had come to a point in my life where I was barely able to get out of bed each day. I could not even do the basic things, like organizing, laundry, cleaning, or managing the mail. I had absolutely no energy, and I began to feel paralyzed.

At the time, I was managing a very large construction project. Though this was the third time I had managed a project of this magnitude and I was accustomed to working very long hours, something felt very different this time.

I was in my fifties, and I was working twelve to sixteen hours a day, so I knew that some of the changes that were happening to me were partly due to exhaustion. After the project was completed, I decided to take some much-needed time off. I was already being proactive about what I was feeling and had started reading books about the importance of adequate high-quality nutrition, the thyroid and other hormones. From what I gathered, I immediately identified with the nutritional and thyroid issues. I went to my husband to confirm some of the symptoms, and he told me, "You have every single one of those issues." And I said, "I know."

I had already been to my general practitioner to have my thyroid tested but, had never looked into nutritional testing. When my thyroid tests came back "within range," I was told there was nothing wrong with me. But I knew instinctively that the results simply weren't telling my whole story. At the time, I was also having issues with night sweats, so I knew I was going through "the change." Needless to say, I was confused and extremely concerned.

Eventually, there was another problem. I was experiencing an increasing ringing in my ears and was waking up in the morning with my left eye bulging. It was significantly larger than my right eye. It was alarming.

I was convinced that my thyroid was the core issue and went to the doctor a second time. Again, the tests came back "normal," and I became very frustrated. I didn't understand why I was being told that nothing was wrong with me when it was painfully obvious that I was suffering. I had even paid $3,000 for a CAT scan of my brain and my eye, and, again, they found nothing wrong with me. And when I went to get my eyeglasses, the optometrist refused to let me get a new prescription or lenses. He correctly sensed, because of my bulging eye, I might have a tumor or a cyst, which is typically the result of a thyroid problem.

I started looking for alternative doctors in my area who were going to look at it from a different perspective, and I found Dr. Shel. She listened to me carefully, and with genuine concern. Clinically, she knew that I had hormonal, nutritional, and thyroid imbalances. She recommended a saliva hormone panel, a detailed thyroid analysis, and an adrenal work-up as well as a nutritional-deficiency testing.

I anxiously waited for the results for three weeks. It seemed like a lifetime. When I went back to get the test results, I was almost in the red on everything, especially in calcium. This was a huge surprise to me. I had been taking 1,200 mg of over-the-counter calcium supplements each day for ten years, but I was extremely deficient in calcium, along with many other vital nutrients. It was very clear that my body was just not absorbing what it needed to, and that I was taking supplements that were simply not professional-grade. Additionally, my thyroid and other hormones were suboptimal. The tests verified that everything was off kilter. My adrenals were not fully functional, especially after many years of working long hours and not sleeping well. When I realized that I was not actually going crazy, I fell apart in Dr. Shel's office. I cannot describe the sense of affirmation and relief I experienced. Now that I knew what was wrong, I could do something about it.

I started a very gradual process of introducing hormones and vitamins into my regimen. I went back for regular checkups, did more follow-up testing, had the thyroid and hormones adjusted as needed, and it was almost textbook. All my vitamin levels came back to normal as a result of taking the medical-grade vitamins and balancing my hormones.

The entire process was particularly confusing, because my thyroid had always been a concern of mine. When I was sixteen, my doctor had prescribed a very low dose of thyroid medication, which I stayed on until I was twenty-eight years old. After moving to another city and finding a new doctor, I was told I no longer needed thyroid medication. Of course, I believed they knew what they were talking about. The doctor had said that I didn't need thyroid medication, so I stopped. It was that simple. From that point forward, I started having allergies. It's like my whole system stopped working properly. And when I was twenty-nine, I had to have a partial hysterectomy.

So when I finally went back on natural hormones, I started with a very gradual dose of natural thyroid, estrogen, progesterone, and testosterone. I started working on the adrenal glands also, and I couldn't believe it. Within the first week, everything changed. I could already tell a huge difference. The changes were very noticeable. Once I started getting back to a place where I felt like myself, I dove even deeper into my nutritional status and was tested for my specific food sensitivities to make sure I was consuming foods that were agreeable with my body. The food-sensitivity testing showed that I was sensitive to almost all of my favorite foods, which was very disheartening to me. But I was committed to the process, and I was very disciplined about what I could and could not eat so my body could be at its best. This made an incredible difference in reducing my bloating, cramping, GI issues, fogginess, and other debilitating symptoms that I hadn't paid much attention to until they started to subside.

I am still working on keeping balance as I age. In the beginning, once I started feeling better, I was elated and started becoming more energetic. I am a very task-oriented person, so I started getting things done. I began to recognize myself again, and I was excited. I never thought that after working so many long hours and being in my fifties that I could take on any new responsibilities or challenges; however, once I began feeling like myself again, I actually went to real-estate school, got my license, and started a new career. There was no way that I could have done that in the shape I was in before. Within five months, I was able to think more clearly and to get back to being myself.

The vast improvements left a permanent impression on me. I wondered how many other women have suffered from lack of information and alternative medical knowledge. How have women dealt with these sorts of misdiagnoses for several decades? I am awestruck at how women were able to go through the physical and emotional changes, similar to what I experienced, prior to integrative medical testing and treatments. After a little while, I started going through an anger stage, and I still deal with that, because I don't understand why I didn't know what my options were. I felt really betrayed by the medical community. Somebody, somewhere along the way should have said, "Look, you're always in the low range, you've got all the classic symptoms of thyroid deficiency, and you were diagnosed and treated many years ago. Let's just try a little bit of thyroid medicine." It seems so simple when the obvious was brought to my attention. I have since learned that once you've been on thyroid medication, it is very unlikely that you're going to get off it.

Now that I have taken control of my well-being, I feel a new path to health has unfolded before me. I feel so encouraged that we're in an age where we can identify what we need to feel well and whole. I am grateful to the integrative physicians that provide the care needed to help guide us on this amazing journey.

After my journey back to wellness was in full swing, my confidence swelled, and the desire to become an advocate for my health became stronger than ever. I learned that it's difficult to trust your instincts when you're not feeling well, and you're working with traditional doctors who perhaps don't see you as an individual. I've known too many women who are told there is nothing wrong with them. It's more common than we want to believe. You just have to listen to your inner self and keep trying until you find the right doctor. It's a lot easier said than done, but it is so essential to be your own advocate.

This is an awakening spiritual journey as well, because you're learning to listen to yourself, to trust yourself, and to believe in yourself. We are raised to have one hundred percent trust in the medical community. But those days are over. I don't have that level of trust in traditional medicine anymore, but its okay. I have made such an important connection to my own body with Dr. Shel's help, and that is priceless. I encourage people to explore the possibilities of integrative medicine. Our bodies, hearts, and spirits are constantly telling us what we need. We just have to listen. In the moment, you may not get the answers you want to hear, but your instincts will never betray you. Today, I am a better person for having fought through this experience. I am now a complete believer in integrative medicine, and I feel you should find the right practitioner. It may take some time, but I feel like more and more doctors will work toward a more holistic approach to healing. Now, I listen more to my inner spirit—my inner voice. I listen to it more than ever before and it never disappoints me. What a remarkable change.

Integrative medicine is based upon the tried and true scientific facts of traditional medicine along with holistic, alternative, approaches to view and treat each patient as an entirely unique individual. This field combines extensive diagnostic testing, holistic variations to treat root causes of symptoms, nutritional supplements, and lifestyle modifications to be successful. To achieve your wellness-oriented goals, you first need a Physician who is willing to combine the appropriate modalities to provide you with unique alternative options to help correct your individual imbalances. As with Lois, it is common to combine various diagnostic tests, such as nutritional testing, hormone testing, and coritsol testing to provide an extensive overview of all areas that need to be addressed based upon the patient's symptoms and test results. More often than not, this approach yields results that are surprising to the patient as it was with Lois' nutritional deficiencies. It is almost an unspoken agreement between the patient and physician that the goals will be reached and ultimately addressed based on the patient's comfort level and speed at which they want to proceed with their transformation.

It is important to understand that integrative medicine does not look at just one option that may be causing symptoms. Instead, quite the opposite is typically true. Integrative physicians are trained to understand the precise and fragile balance between all functions of the body and how they relate to each other. In the best interest of my patients' health and concerns, these balances are explored as deeply as possible. In my experience, patients appreciate this comprehensive, well-rounded approach compared to the traditional skimming over "normal" ranges of labs. This approach avoids the prescribing of several of the same medications, over and over again, to patients who are indeed very unique in their physical makeup and may not need those medications at all.

Until recently, integrative medicine was not as widely sought out and accepted. Patients as well as medical practitioners are taking notice of the increasing trends that point toward growth in this type of care, because the evidence is becoming clear that health issues can be prevented and treated in a more natural way that is in tune with our bodies. By doing so, the natural balance is restored rather than disrupted by many forms of traditional medicine.

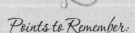

Points to Remember:

- *Consider using your health insurance for major medical expenses, including accidents and other unforeseen emergencies. Consider paying out-of-pocket for preventive health and wellness treatments.*

- *Consider getting tested for your specific nutritional deficiencies, including vitamins, minerals, and antioxidants, and focus on correcting those instead of taking routine vitamins that you "hear or read are good for you."*

- *Stay committed to finding the right doctor who will work with your whole self.*

- *Listen to your inner voice or that "gut feeling" when it comes to your own health. You know your body better than anyone.*

My Vitamin and Supplement Regimen.

What are you taking to support your nutritional status on a daily basis? List your daily intake of nutritional foods and supplements.

_____

_____

_____

_____

_____

_____

_____

_____

_____

_____

_____

_____

_____

_____

_____

_____

_____

_____

_____

_____

_____

_____

_____

_____

_____

_____

THREE:

Journeys to Happiness

*"Most people are about as happy
as they make up their minds to be"*

ABRAHAM LINCOLN

CHAPTER 10:
EAT LIKE YOU LOVE YOURSELF

"If you have health, you probably will be happy, and if you have health and happiness, you have all the wealth you need, even if it is not all you want"

ELBERT HUBBARD

*I*f you are feeling helpless about how to take control of your health, feel reassured by the fact that you can start to feel better almost immediately if you change simple things about your diet. What you eat affects your mood, energy level, weight, immune system, brain function, and even self-esteem. Something as seemingly inconsequential as eating items made with processed sugar every day can have dramatic long-term effects on your body and create an environment for heart disease, diabetes, and high blood pressure.

My patients often ask me, "Dr. Shel, what do you eat?" Personally, I need a lot of energy and stamina to run a busy wellness practice, be a devoted mother, daughter, sister and friend, keep my marriage in great shape, give back to my community and have time for myself. So I have my own eating plan down to a science. Because I am gluten-sensitive, I have developed the following guidelines for myself, which many of my patients also enjoy.

I do not eat:

1. Most white foods, including white rice, white bread, white pasta, white flour

2. Foods containing processed or white sugar or artificial sweeteners (Stevia and Truvia have good research behind them)

3. Beef more than once per week

4. Pork

5. Fried foods

6. Cow's milk

I do eat:

1. Six times a day: breakfast, snack, lunch, snack, dinner, snack

2. Protein with every meal and snack, including chicken, turkey, beans, organic peanut butter, egg whites, lentils, nuts, and more

3. A variety of fresh organic fruits and vegetables throughout the day

4. Almond or rice milk instead of cow's milk

5. Gluten-free oatmeal for breakfast a few times per week

6. Brown rice and quinoa

7. Protein shakes with berries, pea or rice protein and almond milk

I live by an 80/20 rule and recommend it to my patients. It makes the eating program I prescribe for them much less overwhelming and more realistic. This rule for me takes into consideration that 80% of the time I stick to my eating program precisely; 10-20% of the time, however, I allow myself some expected breaks that I may or may not be able to control easily. Sometimes in life, we should all allow ourselves some indulgences that are a part of life and typically a part of important celebrations with family and friends.

Once you get into a rhythm with this sort of meal plan, the way it will make you feel will motivate you to stick with it. You should have your food sensitivities tested to know what you may be reactive to. My favorite labs that you may be able to use through your health insurance provider are Alletess Laboratories, ALCAT, and Immunolabs. Checking your food sensitivities can be a valuable key to help unlock the mysteries of weight gain, lethargy, poor concentration, and several GI issues.

Every day, I see patients who have suffered for years and express that they simply don't feel like themselves. Rarely do they confide in anyone, because women generally are caretakers and give more to others than to themselves. Eventually, these women decide to take matters into their own hands to discover the mystery of why they are experiencing what seems to be a downward spiral of symptoms they can't correct. They begin spending what little time they do have doing their own research, trying to find answers and solutions. Sometimes they are right about what they uncover, but more often than not they can miss a number of other causes that contribute to their state of health, because several root causes can display the same symptoms. That's why testing and diagnosis by an integrative physician is the key to achieving optimal health. ***Pamela's Story***

It hasn't always been easy. But the hardest part of that statement is that I have finally, for the first time in my life, taken full responsibility for my actions and decisions. That's not an easy place to be in. But here I am.

My twenties were the most difficult time of my life. When I was twenty-two, I got married and had my first child. By twenty-eight, I was pregnant with my second child and filing for divorce. That divorce was contentious, nasty, and horrible for everyone involved. It took a huge emotional and financial toll on me and my children. But even with all my hard work and professional aspirations, I had to make more money. I started a jewelry business to create a second income. Obviously, I was stressed out, tired, and worried all the time. Between trying to be the best mom I could be and running a child-care business along with my jewelry business, my entire life was about caring for others. I put my children first and began the slow and unhealthy process of neglecting myself.

A year ago I felt overweight, ugly, and not the slightest bit sexy. It wasn't always like that. I used to feel pretty. But a year ago, I didn't feel like a woman who was desired in anyway. For me, it didn't matter if I weighed one hundred eighty pounds or three hundred eighty pounds—I just didn't feel right. I was upset with myself, because I know that I was responsible for where I was. Nobody forced me to eat the food that I love so much. I had a romance with food. I had a love affair with food. I watched the Food Network and considered myself a total foodie. Even when we went to Las Vegas, we didn't go to gamble—we went to eat.

I grew up with an Italian mother who regularly cooked for twenty. I grew up during the "clean-your-plate" era—you did not get up from the table until you cleaned your plate and bread with every meal. We now understand that people simply can't eat that way, so now it has been a process of reflecting a lot on where I was, and where I am going with my relationship to food.

I knew I needed help. For every positive thing that I was committed to in my life, I was equally committed to sabotaging myself. When I lost two pounds, which would take every ounce of willpower and effort I could muster, I would reward myself with a big piece of luscious cake. I made excuses for myself constantly and continued with the behavior for years. Just prior to seeking the help that gave me the strength to take care of myself for the first time in a long time, something had shifted in me, and I was ready to embrace this new concept of healing with an integrative doctor.

I said to myself, "I don't know how I'm going to do this, but I am doing it." I gathered up my last bit of strength and began to pray for the help to make a major change in my life before I reached thirty-five. I wanted to conquer my demons and finally become the woman I always knew I could be but never had the strength to become. I had tried and failed at so many beginnings up to this point. I wasn't really sure why this time would be different, but there was a very deep part of me that knew my life was about to change. In my mind, I had finally stumbled upon a doctor who was giving me new information about my health, which gave me a renewed sense of hope and determination.

Being the type-A, organized, efficient, in-control person that I am, I had done all my research about weight-loss resistance, so I had already self-diagnosed prior to seeing Dr. Shel. When we sat down to discuss my wellness, I wanted to launch into everything I needed her to do for me. My first priority was to lose the weight, which proved to be an on-going battle regardless of which fad diet I was partaking in at the time. It usually left me astonished and disheartened that it didn't work, so I was convinced that I had food allergies that were keeping me from my ideal weight.

After reviewing my medical questionnaire, it appeared that I was experiencing hormone imbalance, so I agreed to have my levels tested, since thoughts of being premenopausal were running through my head, and I wanted to be sure that I wasn't.

Dr. Shel explained that it was not uncommon for women my age to suffer from hormonal imbalances, primarily relating to progesterone deficiency and estrogen dominance. I already sensed that the level of care I was about to receive was going to far exceed what I had experienced from a general practitioner, an internist, an OB, or an endocrinologist. This was definitely different.

The first order of business was to get hormonally balanced even before I started a weight-loss regimen. This made a lot of sense to me. For the longest time, I thought I had been allergic to some random food, like bananas. In my mind, I thought that if I eliminated some magic combination of foods, my problems would be solved, and the weight would just start melting off—I would finally reach that elusive state of happiness. Looking back on it, it seems so ridiculous, but I find now that it is so common for women. We are always searching for answers to our questions; however, since there is a lack of reputable information out there, we settle with self-diagnosing ourselves or simply living with the way we feel and try to believe there is nothing else wrong with us.

After a few tests, we began to get a very clear picture of what my chemical make-up really was. Hormonally, I was severely out of balance. I received a totally customized program that was unique to my needs, including natural hormones, natural supplements, and healthy lifestyle changes that were well over due. I felt an incredible ease knowing that I might be close to solving the problems that my body was having. While my thyroid seemed to be in the optimal range, bio-identical progesterone was recommended to naturally balance my body. I slowly began to realize that, while my physical goal was to lose weight, I needed to balance my hormones in order to do so and, it would stabilize my moods as well. This made a lot of sense to me.

I always believed that I was basically a happy person by nature. But as my hormones began to change, I realized that my personality, moods, and attitudes were changing beyond recognition. At the beginning of my healing process, I was a basic size twelve. I was not obese, and my husband thought I was beautiful. I was very good at hiding my weight strategically under clothes. I knew that my natural body size was very different from what I was carrying around. It was the way that my body felt that just didn't seem right. Often times I felt *bloated and tired and was craving food that was not good for me. I needed to change all of that.*

I began to dig deep and to take responsibility for the poor choices in my life. And, shockingly enough, it wasn't all about food. It was about a sense of self-worth and the ability to deal with my emotions in real time without hiding behind a comfortable pattern of eating to soothe. This was a particularly difficult part of the journey, because I come from an Italian family full of amazing cooks. When all is said and done, I absolutely love food. I love the sense of family and community that comes from sharing a big meal. I love the ritual of stirring, plating, and sitting down with family and friends who love and appreciate the sensual experience of enjoying food as much as I do. Food brings people together and can be exciting, inviting, and comforting. And after a delicious, lovingly prepared feast, I love that feeling of warmth, fullness, and contentment that is the perfect sedative at the end of a rough day.

So when I began to lose weight, in some respect it might have felt like an indictment against that part of my life. I was absolutely unprepared for one of the most difficult parts of this process—the loss of relationships. As I embarked on this new journey, some of my friends just couldn't relate to me anymore. In retrospect, I think that my friends and I bonded over difficult situations, problems, and misery. But I just wasn't in that place anymore. I felt like I was glowing, and the problems we all had in common had essentially gone away for me. I lost several relationships with women whom I considered my close friends because they always wanted to just keep complaining and not take control of their health and lives. Sadly, they just couldn't be happy for me nor could they understand the new me who was finally in control of her life.

My husband and I now have a different kind of closeness. I think that closeness has come as a result of me wanting something good for myself and then having the strength to follow through on what I need to do to achieve that. I'm not sabotaging myself anymore.

I truly want what is best for my life, which, in turn, is best for my family. And I think he's proud of me for that. And to earn my husband's respect is huge for me. That is something that everyone needs: respect and affirmation from those who love you the most.

Although I am proud of the work I've done to understand my body and to care for it, I do have a lingering regret that I am still struggling with—I have a daughter who will be thirteen this summer, and she struggles with her weight. This is a terrible legacy that I have handed down to her. My grandmother, my mother, I, and now my daughter have all experienced a very complex relationship with our bodies and food. I only wish that I would have taken control of my health before my children were old enough to remember these destructive patterns.

Right now, I have to find a way to help her, and I really believe that some well-guided therapy can help her self-esteem. It is so painful, as a mother, to see your daughter doubt herself so regularly and so profoundly. My daughter is absolutely beautiful both inside and out, and it saddens me to know that I had something to do with her inability to see what so many people see in her. She is wonderful.

How can she not look in the mirror and see how beautiful she is? How could I go so many years seeing and feeling the same thing? I've handed down an attitude, an emotional reflex, maybe even a way of being that cannot be undone easily.

What she has learned is that I used to eat when I was happy or sad or to celebrate. She saw that I ate when things were going well and when things were stressful. She has learned that eating can soothe, preoccupy, or redirect emotions of every kind. In being my daughter, she has learned that something outside yourself—in this case, food—can be used to medicate emotions so you just don't have to deal with them. But what I never explained to her is that the emotions don't go away. They resurface somewhere else and in a much bigger way. When you use food to alter your state of mind or your

*mood, it's just like any other drug. But to be able to face your feelings
as they are happening can help keep you safe, healthy, and happy.
It's about finding a healthy balance. Thank God, I am me again!*

It is quite common for me to consult with patients who
have taken their health into their own hands and have figured
out what is making them experience symptoms that were not
evident before, and I encourage this. However, I also encourage an open mind to treat the body as a whole and to not
focus on just one particular symptom, such as rapid weight
gain, possible diagnosis, or recommended treatment.

Our bodies work with precision and synchronicity to
keep us healthy and full of vitality. If one part of the body
begins to function sub-optimally, the domino effect begins to
cause other areas of the body to do the same. The outcome is
many symptoms that are the direct result of lack of precision
and synchronicity. The goal is not to treat these symptoms
individually but to treat the causes individually and the body
as a whole. Once balance is restored from within, you will
find a renewed sense of being, increased clarity, and you will
have an improved state of mind. You will be able to uncover
underlying issues that have psychologically contributed to
sub-optimal health in the past and find ways to change those
aspects for the future.

Pamela makes a very important point about the message
we are giving to the next generation of women: our daughters, nieces, and granddaughters, as I mentioned previously.

These young women need to see role models of women
who do not always expect perfection from themselves. They
need to know that it is not only okay, but imperative to cherish, honor, and take care of ourselves. We have many roles to
play as women, and we must refill our bucket constantly by
offering time for ourselves, bonding with our loving support-

ers, and balancing our health. What they go through in their lives depends on the paths we leave for them. We as women need to take this responsibility very seriously. I know I certainly do with my daughter, Zoe.

Ask yourself these questions: "Would you want your daughter to live a life of self-sacrifice? Do you want to see her overworking and being completely over stressed just so that she can take care of others and forego her own health"? If the answer is "NO", you and I need to stop modeling that for her. She will certainly follow in our footsteps. Let us lay down a better, more positive path filled with self care and self preservation for the future women in our lives. They deserve it, as do we!

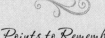

Points to Remember:

- *Focus on eating to live, not living to eat.*

- *Ask yourself the question, "What do I want to role model for the next generation of women—our daughters and granddaughters?"*

- *Live your life the way you want your future generations to live theirs*

- *Remind yourself that food is a healthy and wonderful part of life that should not be abused. Don't punish yourself with "bad" food choices.*

- *Break the emotional eating cycle once and for all.*

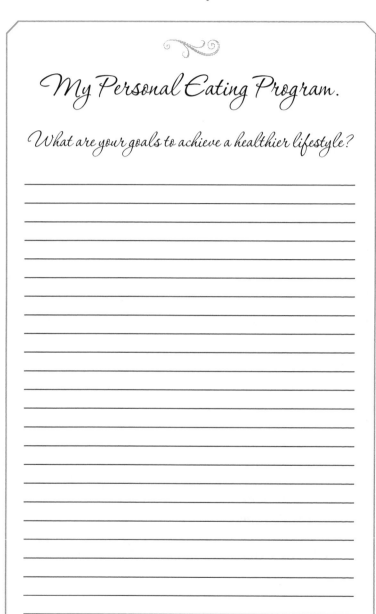

My Personal Eating Program.

What are your goals to achieve a healthier lifestyle?

CHAPTER 11:
THE TRUTH ABOUT AGING

*"The more you praise and celebrate your life,
the more there is in life to celebrate"*

OPRAH WINFREY

*N*ow that I am in my forties, I have a different view about aging than what I believed in my twenties. We are so conditioned in our society to view aging as something to be feared and to be fought. But the work that I do with women emphasizes the importance of not only accepting ourselves at each stage in life, but also celebrating how far we've come. Clarity, wisdom, and peace come with age. I would have given anything to experience this when I was younger. But it was impossible—life experiences, choices, and the evolution of culture all contribute to how well we decide to age. That's right—many of my patients tell me that they realize they are now in charge of the quality of their lives and their *actual* ages, and I commend them for that. It could not be truer.

I see women all the time who say they struggled with self-image when they were younger. They disclose that they continually had issues with their weight, skin, hair, and other areas that made them feel unattractive and fragile. But as they grew older, they learned more about how the female body works and how best to take care of it. The result is a new generation of physiologically empowered women who feel strong, smart, sexy, and most importantly, at peace with themselves.

As you grow older, your life can become more affluent and complete as a result of the people you know, the friends you've made, experiences you've endured, and the successes you've enjoyed along the way. In other words, life can just get better and better as we age. From a medical perspective, women simply do not have to look worse or to feel worse; we can actually look and feel better while significantly slowing the physical aging process. Highly advanced testing, known as Telomere testing by SpectraCell, analyzes an individual's telomere length to determine the person's true chronological age. This, for many of us, is a wake up call when we realize how rapidly we are aging. We are then motivated to take action to slow down this aging process. Chronological aging is something that we can't stop, but how we feel can change and improve beyond measure.

I have patients who have endured extreme stress in their lives, whether it's attributed to their careers, relationships, the many roles they fill in their daily lives, or caring for ill family members. I encourage each and every one of them to take control of their happiness and, most importantly, to take time to lower their stress and to cherish the precious gift of life that was given to them. We are prone to give and give until we are completely worn down, no longer recognize ourselves when we look in the mirror, and feel hopeless and helpless. This can happen to any woman at any age in her life. I encourage all my patients to be gentle with themselves, take the time they need to de-stress, and show themselves the same love they are so committed to giving everything and everyone else in their lives.

Rita's Story

Nine years ago, when my son was a nineteen-year-old college student, he broke his neck in a freak fall off a friend's porch. He stayed in the ICU, and I didn't leave his side. The doctors finally told us that he was partially paralyzed from the neck down and he would be in a wheelchair for the rest of his life. While he had some movement, it was very spotty. The only thing we knew for sure was that it was going to be a long road ahead.

I thought certain responsibilities as a mother were long over, but now I would be worrying about and caring for my grown son all over again. Even though I've always been a strong person, this experience was beyond my comprehension. It was absolutely the lowest point of my life. I don't think I can describe the feeling of complete helplessness and loss that I experienced.

I don't know if anyone can understand the pain, suffering, and sheer exhaustion that experiences like this can inflict on someone. I did not go out for three years after the accident. All I could do was take care of my son. I watched my beautiful, intelligent, vibrant son reduced to having others care for his basic physical needs. I was worried about his mental and emotional states as well as his physical body. It was almost too much to bear.

When someone suffers a spinal injury, the chances of death increase dramatically, and this is how vulnerable my son was. I was constantly in fear of losing him. A mother's most powerful instinct is to protect her child. I fought so hard, every single day, to keep my son comfortable, safe, loved, and, above all, alive.

I worked diligently with rehabilitation experts, doctors, and scientists to get my son to a point where he could take care of himself. But he's still in danger, even though he lives by himself, has a job, and has a girlfriend. The reality is that he is still—and will always be—in a lot of danger.

I've had the hardest time picking myself up after his accident, because it's a tragedy that you are reminded of every single day. I've almost adopted a warrior mentality in order to cope with what has happened. I feel as though I always have to be prepared and I have to be in good health to maintain this role. I also need to have the clarity and strength of mind to deal with this difficult situation every single day.

During that time, I was also going through menopause, and, remarkably, I was doing well emotionally. I was lucky. But, I had a long road ahead of me, and it was extremely important that I be in control of how I was aging. There were things I could do now to keep strong, sane, and focused for my own well-being, but also for the benefit of my son.

I entered a contest that Dr. Shel did for the Houston community for a "Mommy Makeover". She and the judges were so touched by my son's story that I was the lucky winner. God has His ways and I felt like the luckiest person. She gave me a $10,000 INNER & OUTER WELLNESS MAKEOVER! It was like a dream. She wanted to begin with helping me feel revived on the inside first. After completing my saliva and blood tests, Dr. Shel revealed that I did have hormonal imbalances that I wanted to correct immediately so I could begin to take control of how quickly I was aging. I wanted to feel vital, balanced, energetic, and "on my game" once again.

This was the driving desire in me that made me so eager to understand what was happening with my body and to beautify myself in the process. Seeing Dr. Shel for the first time was a bit awe-inspiring. I had been very impressed with how much she seemed to care about people. It was very obvious to me that she was on a mission to help people better their lives. After that first consultation and completion of my tests, I felt very excited about the treatments she suggested and the journey I was about to take.

To assist me with the internal aging process that was taking place, she identified which vitamins I was most seriously lacking by doing a nutritional test called SpectraCell. and gave me a list of customized supplements. She also prescribed a bio-identical hormone regimen with creams and low dose thyroid.

We then decided to address the external aging that was beginning to be noticeable on my face so we moved forward with laser skin tightening, Pearl skin rejuvenation, Botox, and fillers as well as other laser treatments. Growing up in Florida, it was popular to lie out in the sun and tan. We didn't know any better, and my skin took a serious toll. So I was coming to Dr. Shel with major skin damage that I wanted to address.

I have a new-found drive to take care of myself that was compounded by my son's accident. I am fifty-seven years old, and I come from a generation that puts taking care of your family as one of the most important things you can do in life. I have to be sensible and do what I need to do to keep healthy. Because if I fall apart, then part of me believes that my family will fall apart too. I'm just not going to do that to the people I love most. I realize the world doesn't revolve around me, but I do believe that women set a tone in the home that regulates and affects everyone's moods and mind-sets.

I think this also feeds into how people look. In my experience, I can remember instances when people simply responded better to me when I looked nice. I'm not sure why that is, but I do know that I also feel better about myself when I look my best. There are things that I want to do in my life, and I'm not going to let how I look be a barrier to whatever I want to do. Besides, it's fun to look nice. I think that when your face and body look nice, you tend to want to be out in the world more. It's not about vanity—it's about taking the time to care for you and wanting to be engaged in life. When you are faced with unbearable stress, it's a relief to be able to do something for yourself.

I am also a role model for my two sons which makes being kind to yourself absolutely critical. Life can be very challenging, and while we hopefully always have people around who love us, we have to turn to ourselves first to provide that gentle care. I want to teach them, through my own self-care, that they are worthy of the best things in life. I want them to love themselves and to be happy. That is my dream as their mother. You want your children to grow, to be self-sufficient, and to have the emotional maturity and inner resources to make good decisions and to be happy.

As a mother, I saw so many women in my life just give up on themselves once they had children. They would kill themselves making healthy meals for their kids, but they would neglect their own diets and end up gaining weight. Everything would be about the kids. Women are so good at making excuses about why they don't have time to take care of themselves. But what they really need to know is that if they don't, they are setting very poor examples for their children. Children do what their parents do. If you want them to be happy and healthy, you need to be happy and healthy. It's so simple.

I feel so sad for my sister and my friends who, one by one, just gave up on taking care of themselves while they raised children. They would spend all of their money on clothes for the kids while Mom went without. I see this with my sister, who has four children. She was a great mother, but she bent over backwards to give her kids everything, while she neglected herself. Now that her children are grown, they are doing the same thing in their own lives. It's a vicious cycle. Kids are being taught that to love someone is to sacrifice, to suffer, and to not care for you. That couldn't be further from the truth. People that do that eventually will scramble to find ways to comfort themselves and to cope. They turn to food, cigarettes, alcohol, or [bad] relationships. It's sad.

There are so many things that I want to accomplish in my life, and I am gearing myself up to do those things armed with my refreshed skin and balanced body. I want to be active and continue to exercise. In fact, I haven't exercised this much since I was in high school in the 1970s! I'm proud to say that I am in great shape now, thanks to balanced health with Bio-Identical hormones and medical grade nutritional supplements. I have worked hard for that. I joined the YMCA and started taking aerobic dance classes and kickboxing lessons. I feel so much stronger than I have felt in years. The other day I went to the grocery store, and I swung the door open so hard that I thought I was going to rip it off its hinges! It was that moment that made me feel like all of my hard work was paying off. I actually felt like Wonder Woman. I am no longer frail or scared or sad. Sure, I still have those moments, but I can look back on this time in my life and feel so proud that I didn't give up. I managed to face an incredibly heartbreaking situation and figure out a way to stay true to myself. It motivated me to become very clear about who I wanted to be and how I was going to deal with life. Little things don't upset me anymore. Traffic, the mean guy at the post office, the rude phone calls—none of it affects me or matters at all. I am in control of how I feel and respond.

Not only did all the work I did on myself make me healthier, I felt like I was finally having more fun in my life. I wanted to be out in the world. I wanted to participate in life and to embrace my interests and passions. I was trying different things and leaving behind relationships and experiences that were not healthy for me. It seems so obvious, but so much of adopting a healthy lifestyle has to do with choosing food and activities that you really love. You may not like spinach, but if you love squash, eat more of that. You may not like aerobics, but if you like to swim, make that your daily routine. There are always healthy choices that don't seem like a compromise or sacrifice. It just takes a lot of trial and error. I was inspired to go for my dreams and to heal my life. And we're just getting started.

Much like Rita, even in times when your world seems to be on a vicious downward spiral, you can seek the help and encouragement you need, but you have to be at the right place in your life to accept the help. Luckily we are in an era where integrative practitioners are becoming more pre-dominant and widely accepted, which results in your having access to the care that you absolutely need and, more importantly, deserve to achieve optimal health and benefit from anti-aging treatments. Embracing an integrative practitioner can ultimately change your life, as they become your advocate for complete health. They achieve this by taking into consideration all aspects of wellness, which includes: the physical body, emotional status, spiritual quotient, and outward beauty to promote healthy aging. If one of these areas of complete wellness is lacking, then, the "entire" person begins to experience symptoms that are not familiar to them. Thus, begins the downward spiral.

Sometimes we can't give ourselves the love we deserve, so we seek people who can give it to us and teach us how to take good care of ourselves again. This is the type of care you will receive from an integrative physician. He or she will guide you on your path while allowing you to take the steps as slowly or quickly as you desire and only when you are ready and comfortable. Once the first step is taken, life begins to open up to you and to show you its beauty again. At that moment, you can begin to appreciate and relish the fact that you are alive and faced with endless possibilities. I encourage you to take that first step to regain a sense of yourself and the first step in your ascent back up the spiral staircase.

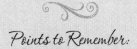

Points to Remember:

- *It is never too late to take control of your inner health and external beauty.*

- *Although we cannot control unforeseen challenges, we can decide how we will respond to and deal with those challenges. (much as my mother did when she lost her 25 year old son)*

- *Be gentle with yourself as you proceed down the path to wellness. You may be the first in your family to break unhealthy habits passed down through generations. Support for you is available.*

My Healthy Aging Plan.

What does the term "healthy aging" mean to you?

How are you going to remain healthy while you age?

PART FOUR:

Journeys to Harmony

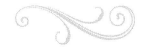

*"Happiness is when what you think,
what you say and what you do are in harmony"*

MAHATMA GANDHI

CHAPTER 12:
CHALLENGING TRADITIONAL MEDICINE

"Judge your success not just by what you have accomplished, but by the person you have become"

RANJANA CLARK

According to the American Holistic Medicine Association, "holistic medicine is the art and science of healing that addresses the whole person—body, mind, and spirit". The practice of holistic medicine integrates conventional and alternative therapies to prevent and treat disease and, most importantly, to promote optimal health. Good health, from a holistic standpoint, is therefore defined as the unlimited and unimpeded free flow of life force energy through our bodies, mind, and spirit.

Holistic medicine encompasses all safe and appropriate modalities of diagnosis and treatment. It includes analysis of physical, nutritional, environmental, emotional, spiritual, and lifestyle elements. Holistic medicine focuses upon patient education and participation in the healing process."

The Principles of Holistic & Integrative Medical Practice

Holistic physicians are dedicated to providing and promoting a variety of safe, effective options in the diagnosis and treatment of the entire person, including education for lifestyle changes and self-care and alternatives to conventional drugs and surgery.

Searching for the underlying causes of disease is preferable to treating symptoms alone. *Holistic & Integrative physicians expend as much effort in establishing what kind of patient has a particular disease as they do in establishing what kind of disease a particular patient has.* This is a very notable point, because, more often than not, many people are predisposed to certain diseases and ailments genetically. They may alter their habits, their stressors, their attitudes, and their psyches due to those risks. Additionally, integrative physicians emphasize prevention over treatment. Focusing on prevention offers many advantages, including improved long-term physical health, mental well-being, and financial health. Preventive care is certainly more cost-effective in the long run, and is much gentler to the body. Integrative practitioners view illness and disease as a reflection of imbalances and dysfunction in the whole person; diagnoses are not just based on isolated symptoms. In the view of many doctors like me, optimal health goes far beyond the absence of sickness. It is the presence of a true state of health, happiness, and harmony.

Healing depends so much on the sincere and trusting relationship that develops between the patient and the physician. Well-trained integrative doctors rely heavily on the conversations they have with their patients. They encourage their patients to be advocates for their own health and to be knowledgeable about how various protocols are affecting them. It is a partnership of healing based on the unique needs of the patient and the specialized training of the physician. In that respect, it is critical that physicians themselves should be a model of health, wellness, and self-care for their patients.

Integrative practitioners fully understand the healing powers of positive thinking, humor, hope, and, most importantly, love. These feelings have an amazingly divine power to help neutralize an environment of toxicity that comes with feelings of depression, fear, worry, anger, loss, shame, or grief. Unconditional love is the most powerful healing force in the world. Physicians who choose an integrative and holistic approach to healing use this kind of love as their primary tool. They have compassion for patients, love for themselves, and respect for other practitioners. Unfortunately, many people simply stop honoring and loving themselves when they don't feel they are in a complete state of wellness and health. It is my personal mission to heal patients by providing them with natural treatments to resolve the causes of their symptoms while giving them the tools that allow them to love and to give to themselves again. This will gradually instill an improved state of wellness in them.

All too often, I hear stories about health-care treatments that went wrong due to the patient not being treated as an individual and the physician not delving deep enough to uncover the causes of abnormal life-changing symptoms. This was the case with Suzy before she came to see me. I was able to gain her trust by letting her know that my goal was to see her as a unique woman, not just another patient with symptoms that are similar to others.

Suzy's Story

When I was only in my early twenties, I began experiencing extremely heavy and multiple periods every month—so heavy that I would consistently bleed throughout most of the month. No matter what I did, they just seemed to be getting worse and worse. I was overwhelmed and felt completely out of control of my life. My OB-GYN put me on every possible birth control in order to regulate my menstrual cycle, but nothing worked. At the same time, I was going through dramatic mood swings, and I just didn't feel like I was in my right mind. After numerous visits to my doctor, he recommended a very serious treatment plan—chemical menopause (very strong chemicals to stop the periods but [leaving] many undesirable side effects). Here I was, only twenty-two, and my doctor was telling me that I had to undergo menopause in order to stop my severe bleeding. At the same time, one of my other doctors prescribed strong psychotropic medications for what he believed to be a bipolar disorder due to the severe mood swings. At that age, despite telling him that I did not believe that was the problem, I respected the doctor's opinion and underwent treatment anyway.

The chemical menopause was emotionally very traumatic but seemed to reduce my menstrual symptoms and mood swings. But for twelve years, I continued to be on heavy psychotropic medications, thinking the mood swings were caused by my so-called bipolar label. The diagnosis of bipolar disorder never seemed to fit me, and I learned that even having that diagnosis was a major stigma. Friends, family, even colleagues treated me differently, and I lost friends, relationships, and opportunities due to the diagnosis. I felt like an outsider—someone to stay away from or to fear and to be avoided. I was unsure of myself, confused and alone with this uneasy feeling that I wasn't exactly what my doctors said I was.

Under the proper definition, bipolar disorder (also known as manic-depressive illness) is characterized by periods of high-energy, manic behavior alternating with periods of low-energy, depressive behavior. These two extremes are typically bridged by normal behavior most of the time. I knew in my heart that I was not suffering from a mental disorder. My system felt out of alignment, but I didn't know what to do. I had a gut feeling that the heavy bleeding in my twenties was somehow related to my mood swings. I just knew in my heart that I was not bipolar. I am a counselor by training and started out as a crisis counselor. I see many clients with bipolar disorder – and my symptoms were not the same. If someone would've spent the time they needed to really know who I was while keeping an open medical mind, perhaps they would see that as clearly as I did. My mother and I had always thought that I might be suffering from serious hormonal issues, but the doctors never seemed concerned or willing to delve into the deeper possibilities.

By the time I reached my mid-thirties, something even more alarming began to happen. I was experiencing extremely sharp pains behind my eyes, and I was suddenly going blind. Doctors said that I might be having glaucoma or stroke-like symptoms. One of the doctors determined that this was caused by the side effects of the psychotropic meds and advised me to get off the meds to see if that would help.

During that time, I became even more determined to find out the causes for my various health problems and to try more natural and organic methods. I began researching doctors who specialized in hormone imbalances and found Dr. Shel. I immediately underwent a series of hormone and nutrition and food-sensitivity testing. The results were conclusive. I had severe nutritional deficiencies, and my hormones were very unbalanced. I had extremely low progesterone and estrogen levels. My FSH (Follicle Stimulating Hormone) level was in the menopausal range. At thirty-eight, I was going through premature menopause. I was in shock and very upset that all these years, no other doctor caught it. My chances of becoming a mother without dramatic infertility treatments were essentially over.

I began a treatment regimen that included a new nutritional program and bio-identical hormones. Within only a few months, I was a different person. I was sleeping soundly, more energetic, less anxious, and, most importantly, I was truly happy and peaceful for the first time in many, many years. I was no longer experiencing any symptoms related to menopause or the bipolar diagnosis I had been enduring for so long. But getting well and finally identifying what was truly presenting problems for me was very bittersweet.

At thirty-nine years old, I am still struggling with the pain and anger of undergoing chemical menopause, being on psychotropic drugs that I did not need, and experiencing permanent damage to my vision as a result of those drugs.

I am a counselor (LPC) by profession, and now I encourage people who come to me for help to research nutritional deficiencies/food allergies and hormonal testing. I encourage them to consider working with medical professionals who understand, honor, and respect the whole person. I am now a passionate advocate for questioning serious diagnoses that could change the course of a person's life forever. I believe that the current health-care system should be challenged in every possible way. If enough women stand up for more comprehensive health care, we may be able to make a change for future generations.

I have to believe that I went through this experience in order to help other people. I found a sense of strength and purpose during this process that I never thought I could have. The most important thing I learned was how important it is to simply love yourself enough to fight for your health, your dignity, and your future.

As in Suzy's story, many women have dealt with misdiagnoses and a negative label that they have had to carry in regards to their physical and/or mental condition. I encourage you to take the time and patience to be your own advocate and take control of your well-being by conducting your own research and consulting with as many doctors as you need to until you feel a sense of comfort with one or with a group of them. After all, it is your body, and no one knows it better than you. Trust in yourself, your intuition, and your instinct. A compassionate doctor who listens to you, and is in sync with your needs, can indeed put you on the right path to wellness, without harming your body.

When it comes to psychotropic medications, please make sure that you are on them because you truly need them by getting more than one opinion. I would encourage you to also consider getting an opinion from at least one Integrative physician before starting on a treatment regimen that includes psychotropic medications, surgery, or treatments that you are not comfortable with. This will allow you to look at the "whole" picture. As a fellow practitioner once very accurately said, "there is no-one that has a deficiency in Prozac, Zoloft or any other anti-depressant." Remember this before you take your next antidepressant or anxiolytic drug. Please be sure that all your true deficiencies are first corrected – whether they are of hormones, thyroid, nutrients, antioxidants, or minerals. Be sure that you are reducing your stress, and engaging in yoga, meditation, or other breathing exercises. Attempt to work on a healthy eating program with nutrient rich, organic foods if possible. Enroll yourself in a regular moderate exercise program which includes resistance exercises. Revive your body with at least seven to eight hours of sleep per night. Surround yourself with loving, positive people who give you a true support system. Finally, and most importantly, love yourself for the beautiful, amazing person that you are. See the BEST in yourself and give the BEST to yourself. You deserve it!

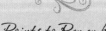

Points to Remember:

- *Mental illness is a serious physical condition that should be identified and treated. However, many times patients with hormonal imbalances, food allergies, or nutritional deficiencies are misdiagnosed with mental illnesses.*

- *Finding a doctor who will test for conditions ,that other doctors do not typically test for, is the first step in narrowing down to a proper diagnosis. Without that, accurate treatment is virtually impossible.*

- *Nobody has a deficiency in antidepressants or anxiolytics. The symptoms of depression may be a direct result of hormonal or nutritional deficiency and/or stress.*

My Personal Health Care Advocates.

Who understands you and supports you with your healthcare needs?

_____

_____

_____

_____

_____

_____

_____

_____

_____

_____

_____

_____

_____

_____

_____

_____

_____

_____

_____

_____

_____

_____

CHAPTER 13:
GETTING SLEEP, ACHIEVING HARMONY

"A good laugh and a long sleep are the best cures in the doctor's book"

IRISH PROVERB

One of the primary complaints that women share with me is the experience of feeling "cloudy", "out of sorts", and "unfocused". Women who were once extreme multi-taskers and incredible organizers suddenly find it difficult to remember simple things, and lose their entire train of thought. Certainly, this experience can be scary and unnerving to someone who has prided herself on her competence, dependability, and intelligence.

But losing focus is a normal and very common problem that many women experience. This symptom may be part of a larger problem stemming from a variety of imbalances, and can be easily treated. Lack of focus may be misdiagnosed as depression, stress, or extreme fatigue. But the reality is that sleep deprivation, imbalances in nutrients and hormones such as estrogen, testosterone, cortisol, thyroid, progesterone, or other hormones, may be contributing to "foggy thinking," as some of my patients describe it.

Eventually, this mental cloudiness makes it even more difficult for women to seek the medical attention they desperately need. They talk themselves out of engaging in healthy behaviors or simply seeking help of any kind. They are convinced that how they feel is "all in their heads"; but the symptoms are real. Although traditional doctors may dismiss being unfocused as a natural sign of aging, I believe that mental clarity is a better natural state, which one must strive to achieve. Once you are thinking clearly, it is even more likely that you'll make healthier choices that will dramatically improve the quality of your life. With mental clarity, you are more likely to make better food choices, to exercise more regularly, to seek emotional support as needed, and ultimately to restore the harmony that can quickly be whisked away without the appropriate life choices and balance.

Kyra's Story

I was in a fog. And it was serious. I had always considered myself an organized, self-assured, and highly reliable person. Now, something was different. At forty-five, I was a successful physical therapist and educator. I had always prided myself on being fit, active, and in control of my body. With no history of depression in my own life or in my family, I began to panic about what was happening to my psyche at this point in my life.

I had always been somebody who could remember everything. This is something I prided myself on, and a trait that I was known for both personally and professionally. I always had a mental checklist in my mind. I could remember dates and numbers, and people whom I had talked to and specific details about them. But I had gotten to the point that if I had thought about something and if I didn't act on it or write it down immediately, it was gone in the flash of a second. I would think of something to do, and I would get up to go do it, and I would be halfway across the room and think, "Okay, what am I doing, what am I going after?" I would completely lose my train of thought.

As a proactive woman, I had been a successful public speaker and regularly gave presentations as a part of my career and my calling. I enjoyed inspiring, educating, and motivating people, but the changes I was facing began to dramatically undermine my ability to accomplish what I loved most about my job. There were times when I would be giving presentations, and I would completely lose my train of thought and have no idea what I was saying or what point I was trying to make. It would take me several minutes in front of the room (while covering it up very well) to figure out where I was going with a particular idea. It was very disturbing. This was not who I was. I told myself that people like me don't have this kind of problem. I didn't have memory losses or lapses, and so it was something that was very disconcerting for me. I was worried. Additionally, I had also been gaining weight, losing hair, experiencing insomnia, and had skin issues. Overall, I just felt like I was falling apart.

I became so concerned that I began to aggressively research a variety of neurological disorders. I had started doing research online about memory loss, and at that point I started finding research on hormonal imbalances and thyroid conditions. In order to feel some sense of control, I created a checklist and began scouring my memory for things I had learned as a health-care provider and physical therapist. I started to remember lessons I had learned about nutrition and biochemistry and began the process of putting the pieces together.

Because of the concerns I uncovered in my research, I scheduled an appointment with my general practitioner right away. I indicated that I believed my condition may have something to do with my thyroid or possibly a hormonal imbalance. I even talked to my OB-GYN. Of course, they did some routine tests, drew blood, and decided to go forward with specific thyroid testing. Every time my test results came back, the findings were "normal" and "within range." Nothing was wrong. They said, "Maybe you're just depressed and anxious about something, or maybe you just have too much stress in your life." They tried to give me antidepressants but I declined. I was not convinced. This explanation never rang true for me. I did not show signs of depression, and the only thing I was anxious about was the fact that I could not remember even the simplest things. I had always had some level of stress in my life due to the nature of my business, but that had not changed dramatically in the recent past, and neither had my eating or exercise habits. I knew there was something else going on. It was around that time that I crossed paths with Dr. Shel at a professional event. When she shared her philosophy with me, I knew I needed to be her patient. I was lost, and I needed help.

I was forty-five and very afraid. The truth was I hadn't had a full night's sleep in twenty-three years. I truly went more than two decades without proper sleep. When I came to visit Dr. Shel for the first time, I think she sensed my fear, and together we immediately began to explore what was really going on.

That initial meeting came as a complete relief to me, because I literally thought that I was having some sort of a psychological breakdown. I kept saying to myself that, perhaps, I was just making too much of this. Everybody in my life was saying, "Oh, it's just no big deal, you're probably going into perimenopause, everybody goes through this." But I kept thinking that there has got to be a better answer. I just couldn't accept that this was the way it was going to be. I just didn't want to feel this way anymore. I didn't want to snap at my children, yell at my husband, and just have this overwhelming feeling of anger all the time. I committed to myself that I was going to find a solution and I didn't have to feel this way.

When Dr. Shel and I met, we discussed taking more of a holistic approach to improving my health. I was not interested in getting a slew of drugs designed to counteract symptoms. We need to explore all my options. My emotional and psychological states were being stretched thin, and even my marriage was beginning to suffer.

It was kind of like we were living together, but there wasn't the romance we once had. It just wasn't there. It was a very cold relationship, and I wasn't interested in having sexual relations at all. It's hard for me to admit, but there was even one point when I thought if I never have sex again in my life, that would be just fine. Emotionally, for our relationship, it wasn't healthy, because I wasn't holding up my end of the deal in our relationship. I didn't feel happy, vibrant, and certainly not sexy. I felt numb. The changes in my body and mind were also affecting my relationships with my children. They were strained, unpredictable, and fueled by anger.

It was such a difficult time, because I felt like I could not control my emotions. I would constantly lose patience with my children, and they didn't deserve that. It was almost as if I expected perfection from them, because I just had no tolerance. It was very stressful, and everybody in the house could feel it. I had good days, and I had really, really bad days. One of the things that my husband said after I got into Dr. Shel's Wellness program was that he was so thankful to get his wife back. It was as though he and I had both lost the "REAL ME" for some time.

I initially began on thyroid medication and also started bio-identical hormones. My tests indicated that I had subclinical hypothyroidism with low thyroid activity, and my hormones were so imbalanced that some of them barely registered on the scale. I also began taking nutritional supplements based on my individual deficiencies that Dr. Shel had tested for. She then placed me on a specific protocol for my hair and skin, which included zinc, biotin and other B vitamins.

Dr. Shel was emphatic about my sleep patterns needing to improve. She said that adequate sleep was just as important as building up my body with the proper supplements and natural hormones. She recommended that I get at least 7-8 hours of sleep each night. I hadn't given myself this much needed rest in over 2 decades. I attribute this to continually making the excuse that I was simply too busy and had to accomplish too much at the end of the day. Allowing myself the adequate sleep I so desperately needed, gave my body the chance to fully re-

store itself each night. Little did I know that inadequate sleep can lead to serious health issues since this is the time when our body repairs all of the damages from the day be it: emotional, physical, or spiritual stress.

After approximately 6 to 8 weeks of being compliant with my treatment and recommendations, I felt a dramatic difference in every possible way. I even began losing weight, eventually dropping a total of thirty-four pounds. I was on a fast track to returning to my vibrant self.

Now, I have the energy that I'm used to, as well as thick hair, even and moist skin, and a beautiful physique. I have energy and enthusiasm for life, my family, and my business. Mentally, I feel like I am in my twenties and early thirties. I feel like I'm attractive and sexy now, which has been life-changing and has improved my marriage significantly.

Being a health-care practitioner myself, I know that the health-care system wants to be able to test things. But what I've learned is that in traditional medicine, the range of what they say is "normal" for the thyroid and other hormones is an excessively wide range. Apparently. Dr. Shel has discovered through her research and working with thousands of women hat there is a much, much smaller range that is really healthy and optimal. I think that there are probably a significant percentage of women who are wrongfully prescribed antidepressants or mood medications. Women would be much happier, all across the country, if they were actually treated with this newer information. Women need to be treated comprehensively and holistically with attention to nutrition, bio-identical hormones, healthy lifestyle changes, and adequate SLEEP.

Kyra's story represents many different women today. Because of the state of the overall health care and managed care industries and the desire for ultimate cost-effectiveness, doctors may not always consider the whole person. After being a part of this way of practicing medicine and treating my patients for over 13 years, I knew that I could do more for them.

I no longer desired to simply put a band-aid on the causes of their symptoms. Many traditional physicians address their patients' conditions with mainstream medications and never get to their root causes. I know this well because that's how I too was trained and practiced in the past. When I decided to turn to integrative medicine to truly improve the health of my patients, I knew that my desire to practice medicine my way and the overall health of my patients, would both be fulfilled. I embraced the concept of treating the whole patient, not just their symptoms. I managed to do what I hope more women across the U.S. and the world will do in the next decade. I was vigilant about understanding all of women's options and committed to creating a highly personalized program that would keep women happy, healthy, and fulfilled.

I can honestly say that the road a lot of women are on will lead to serious depression, relationship issues, significant weight gain, and poor health, which can, in turn, lead to even more complications, including heart disease and cancer. Countless women have a history in their family of heart problems, diabetes, and high cholesterol, and that is a very dangerous road. Because of the intervention that is now available, many women are on a very different path. I feel as though women have the ability to control their own health now. As a result, they can have the energy, clarity, and desire to focus on themselves in order to be healthy and in complete harmony within themselves. This is after all, what was meant for each of us in our lives.

The bottom line is that women should not be satisfied with the procedures and limitations of traditional medicine. Don't be satisfied with countless prescriptions and shallow examinations by professionals who simply don't have the time, energy, or motivation to know who you really are. Women, no matter what age, deserve to have what they need to feel happy and healthy—without exceptions.

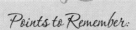

Points to Remember:

- *Don't be a work martyr. Guard your sleep like you would your sight or your hearing.*

- *Sleep at least 7 to 8 hours per night. Sleep health is an integral part of maintaining balance, concentration, and fighting disease. It is investment in yourself and your happiness!*

- *Use your family's health history as an incentive to pay attention to your own well-being. Don't be frightened of the genes they've inherited.*

- *Once you realize your predispositions, you can overcome even overwhelming health challenges with the correct information, guidance, and caring support.*

My Sleep & Relaxation Plan.

What can you do to designate your personal relaxation time every day? How will you schedule 7 to 8 hours to sleep every night?

_____
_____
_____
_____
_____
_____
_____
_____
_____
_____
_____
_____
_____
_____
_____
_____
_____
_____
_____
_____
_____
_____

PART FIVE:

The Healing Begins

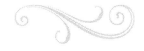

*" Life is like a mirror.
Smile at it and it will smile back at you"*

PEACE PILGRIM

CHAPTER 14:
SPIRITUALITY & HEALTH

*"Learn to relax. Your body is precious,
as it houses your mind and spirit.
Inner peace begins with a relaxed body"*

NORMAN VINCENT PEALE

I'll be honest—I wasn't always certain about my willingness to be open about my spiritual beliefs. As a doctor, the scientific approach to life is encouraged, rewarded, and even celebrated. In Western cultures, doctors typically keep issues of faith to themselves. But in Eastern cultures, the spirit is powerfully integrated into everyday life and work. Faith, religion, spirituality, tradition, and customs of every kind provide powerful and consistent punctuation to lives. That's the way it has always been, and that's why I feel comfortable sharing my story and being exactly who I am.

I believe that the soul is the center of life. If your soul is suffering, your body and mind are quick to follow. The soul needs to be nurtured just like your body needs to be maintained and cared for with proper nutrition, a variety of foods, and clean water. Your soul needs consistent replenishment with time in nature, good thoughts, prayer, meditation, or any of the creative arts. We need food for the body and food for the soul *every single day* to reach a state of optimal well-being.

In the grand scheme of things, the body and soul complement one another completely and beautifully. As a result, absolutely no conflict exists between science and spirituality. With equal attention to each, the body and soul effortlessly help each other to continuously evolve and heal.

As a scientist, I believe all the functions of the body have physical explanations. I also believe in the overwhelming beauty of science's capacity to provide deeper explanations and understandings of God's work. I believe in the mystical power of a conscious universe and in the continuing ability of human beings to discover new explanations for God's creativity on Earth. Like some of the great mathematicians and physicists of our time, I also think that math and science are important aspects of God's unique and powerful language.

But even beyond science, the question arises regarding how spirituality influences emotional and psychological health. As we are now coming to understand, our emotions and psyches are simply extensions of our physical states. Women are particularly self-critical, and spirituality can be a lifeline to managing our respective worlds. Beginning to understand our uniqueness and how important we all are in the dance of life begins with raising our consciousness to new levels, and bridging the gap between the physical world and the spiritual realm.

This new consciousness is a perfect foundation for a deep sense of love and peace. It all begins with the most sacred gift we possess in our lives: **breath**. Without it, we could not be alive. What do you think about when you hear the phrase "take some deep breaths"? Sometimes we are trying to calm down, to take a moment, and to reassess a challenging situation. Sometimes we literally take deep breaths before we go under water in an effort not to drown; or we are simply trying to get from one end of the pool to the other in the quickest, most efficient way. But when we come up, invariably, we are tired, gasping for breath.

Deep breaths connect us to life-giving oxygen as well as to the present moment. So I say that it's important not only to take deep breaths when we are in crisis or trying not to drown (literally and figuratively) but, also, to train ourselves to be conscious enough throughout the day.

Many of my patients say that they don't have the time or energy to simply be with themselves and to pay attention to their own needs at any given moment. But with regular "deep-breath" breaks, we are allowing ourselves the opportunity to do several important things for ourselves: (1) reconnecting with the now and feeling "what is" rather than "what was" or "what will be"; (2) giving our bodies a moment to rest and to integrate the physical experiences of the day—we feel our heartbeats, notice whether we are hungry, tired, or dehydrated, and relax our muscles for some much-needed down time; (3) reducing carbon-dioxide levels in the bloodstream.

For patients who do not practice deep breathing often enough (which is most of us), we can experience decreased oxygen levels and increased health problems. However, when people do practice deep breathing, as a result of richly oxygenated cells, they witness a decrease in common health complaints such as: stress, fatigue, and lack of mental clarity. Many Fortune 500 companies enroll their CEOs in deep-breathing workshops to help them reduce stress in the workplace and improve performance.

I find that even amidst my very busy day seeing patients and pouring all of me into helping them in their challenges,

I take a 2-5 minute break, close my eyes and take some long, deep breaths and focus inward. I highly recommend this exercise no matter what kind of work you do – whether you are a high-powered executive, a caretaker, a service provider or a mom. This exercise will help you not only get through the day, but to enjoy, cherish and maximize your potential for the day. Try it!

We are all special people. We all had different sets of gifts bestowed upon us when we were born. This makes other people, relationships, and life more interesting and less like what we would experience day in and day out if we were all carbon copies of each other. Yet sometimes we continue to find ourselves more interested in what others were gifted with in their lives, and we become overtaken with desire to be like them and to have what they have. In this process, we become more focused on others rather than ourselves. As a result, we never end up fully appreciating the beautiful people that we are, and what we have to offer ourselves as well as to each person we encounter. It has become more and more common for us to not appreciate ourselves, because we think we are not whole, which can be based on believing, "I am not this or that," or "I don't have these things and therefore I am not enough." If we take the time to look into the mirror and truly see ourselves for who we are, we will find that our gifts *are* truly abundant and should be appreciated even if they don't match what we believe others have.

Cultivating everyday spirituality helps us look into ourselves, reflect on who we are, remember all our accomplishments (no matter how big or small), take pride in "mistakes" that made us stronger, and love ourselves. *Remember this mindset* as you begin to overcome your physical obstacles. If you learn to truly love yourself, as we were each meant to, you will have achieved that harmonious and powerful unconditional love that is your birthright.

My Personal Plan For Greater Spirituality.

What are your spiritual beliefs? What can you do to become closer to your true spiritual self?

_____

_____

_____

_____

_____

_____

_____

_____

_____

_____

_____

_____

_____

_____

_____

_____

_____

_____

_____

_____

_____

_____

_____

CHAPTER 15:
TAKING THE FIRST STEP

"The greatest wealth is health"

VIRGIL

*A*s women discover increased health-care options, they will naturally become their own advocates and demand better, more comprehensive care that reflects a more holistic approach. This paradigm shift is absolutely inevitable. Even today, many American families cannot afford the price of traditional health care and intuitively understand that prevention will save not only money, but lives.

Certainly, there will be a lot of reluctance to change, because the initial cost to care for patients holistically requires that the physician spend more one on one time with each patient. That's just a fact.

I am certain that studies will reveal that the long-term costs of not addressing the whole patient will ultimately be several times higher, and that preventive medicine will definitely save money and resources in the long run. The greatest shift in the medical community will be the amount of time doctors are allowed to spend with patients. This is critical. Before insurance companies called the shots, doctors routinely used their discretion to determine the appropriate amount of time to spend with patients. A doctor had the time to ask such questions as, "So, what's going on in your personal life right now?" or "How's the job going?" or "Tell me more about your sleep history. Let's go back to before you were pregnant. Let's see if we can figure this out." But today, routine doctor visits typically run about ten to fifteen minutes. Complaints are determined, a form is filled out, a couple of questions are asked, and a prescription is written.

The patients who generously shared their stories in this book described incidents in doctors' offices that are all too common. A patient is weary, depressed, uncomfortable, dejected, and confused. But, more often than not, that patient is simply told, "Your tests are within normal range. There's nothing wrong with you." But all over the world and throughout history, women have banded together to talk about their bodies and to create remedies and solutions to help heal one another. Generations of women have turned to the natural world, and to tried and true protocols, to assist them in managing their own care and the care of their children. Yoga has been a health mainstay in the Indus Valley and around the world for centuries, promoting flexibility, blood flow, and oxygenation.

Over the centuries, healing remedies have been developed around the world simply based on what works and what doesn't. Probiotics, melatonin, fish oil, omega-3 fatty acids—these are remedies that occur naturally.

For example, the native Khoisan and South African settlers have used red bush tea for centuries to ease the effects of the sun. A cup of red bush replaces body fluids vital to muscular function and cardiac stability that are lost in perspiration. Chinese pharmacies still offer a wide range of herbal and natural remedies alongside modern pharmaceuticals. In

New Zealand, Maoris discovered the healing ability of honey made from flower essences of the Manuka tree. Manuka honey is recommended to fight infections and to overcome stomach bugs.

Now, we have the power of technology and science to help aid the evolution of medicine, but we are squandering these resources by approaching healing from a traditional perspective. The primary focus is on the symptom and the medicine to alleviate that particular symptom. But, as a board-certified physician, I have first-hand knowledge of how the body is affected by the mind. As a spiritual person, I can take it a step further and suggest that it is a beautiful and unique part of the human journey to achieve alignment between the mind, body, and spirit. In many ways, achieving this balance and alignment is our job as human beings. We are more than just people working nine to five, keeping houses, and having families. We can usually meet these basic obligations, but they don't represent the whole story. No, the true role of a human being is to achieve the mystical and divine alignment between body, mind, and spirit. When imbalance exists, so does suffering.

So how do you find a doctor to meet your particular needs? First and foremost, begin with your current doctor. Start an open and direct dialogue about your needs and concerns. Explain to this doctor that you are beginning to understand the link between your mind, body, and spirit, and ask whether he or she feels that exploring that link is important to managing your health. Here is a list of questions that might ignite that important first conversation:

1. *What is your view about the connection between the mind, body, and spirit?*

2. *How much time can I have with you to discuss my concerns?*

3. *Do you test for hormonal imbalances using a variety of tests, including blood and saliva?*

4. *What are your thoughts regarding testing for food allergies and sensitivities that might be contributing to my current symptoms?*

5. *Are you willing to adjust my treatment if I am not experiencing relief within two weeks?*

6. *How often do you prescribe antidepressants? Do you try other treatments before resorting to this?*

7. *Do you believe in nutritional supplements? How would you determine what an individual needs? What brands do you recommend?*

8. *Would you be open to my suggestions in the care of my body?*

9. *Do you look at the "whole person," or do you only deduce your diagnoses and treatment plans based on test results?*

10. *Do you offer referrals for natural weight-loss programs and dietary counseling?*

Chances are that traditional physicians may not meet your current needs. In that case, you can begin the eye-opening process of finding a doctor who can offer the help and hope you need to get started on your path to wellness.

Here are some tips to help you find the doctor who is right for you:

1. *If you have friends or family members who are fit, healthy, and happy, find out if someone close to you is already getting help from a doctor specializing in integrative medicine and wellness.*

2. *Search online for doctors in your community who describe themselves and their practices with such words as "holistic healing," "integrative medicine," "wellness practice," and*

"mind/body/spirit." Do your research to make sure you are working with a board-certified physician who has embraced modern wellness practices.

3. *Get referrals from other wellness professionals, such as: chiropractors, naturopathic doctors, nutritionists, yoga instructors, and others.*

4. *Contact doctors who regularly write about integrative medicine and wellness practices or appear in the media. If they are not taking patients, they often have a network of colleagues who they can readily recommend.*

Once you've narrowed down a handful of prospects, schedule an appointment with the first one your instinct suggests. Get to know that doctor. It is important to find someone with whom you "click" and with whom you feel totally comfortable revealing the details of your life. You need to feel assured that you can confide the details of your physical, emotional, spiritual, and psychological well-being with your physician. This is crucial as honesty is a cornerstone for your doctor-patient relationship, and is crucial for him / her to make proper diagnoses and recommend treatments. Evaluate that doctor by how you "feel" after the visit. Do you feel encouraged, heard, and uplifted, or do you feel hopeless and helpless?

Now it's decision time. At this point, be open to making a life-changing investment in your health that not only will strengthen and lengthen your own life, but will allow you to live, love, and laugh like never before. Additionally, the most cost-effective way to manage your life is to make that important investment in yourself *now*.

My Goal to Find an Integrative Practitioner.

What steps will you take to improve your health with the help of a qualified integrative practitioner?

CHAPTER 16:
STAYING WITH YOUR TREATMENT

*"Take care of your body.
It's the only place you have to live."*

JIM ROHN

es, I realize I am using a tried and true medical term when I say "treatment." But after considering it, I would encourage you dissect the word "treatment" and think of it this way: Treat-me-(n)icely-(t)oday. That's right. Think of the word "treatment" as "treat me nicely today." You should stick with this protocol every single day. One of my patients set up a unique basket system in her bathroom after receiving her treatment protocol, which included nutritional supplements, bio-identical thyroid medication, adrenal support, and progesterone cream. She cleared her shelves and put these items into one basket. In another basket, she put her new natural skin-care products. In the third basket, she put a fresh supply of beautiful mineral-based make-up. Yes, this seems very simple. But because she worked from home, this patient previously had absolutely no routine in the morning other than washing her face, putting her hair in a ponytail, and taking some ibuprofen. Now, she was committed to using the items in those three baskets every single day before she left her bathroom. Steps that are obvious for some women are the humble beginnings of new self-care routines for others.

Research suggests that it takes forty days to establish a new routine or to break a bad habit. You have to commit to forty days to begin to see real and positive change in the right direction.

Staying with treatment and maintaining compliance is an emotional process for many women. You will experience moments when you feel that you've turned a corner and you are "fixed." Many women report to me that once they begin to see improvements in their health and overall well-being, they simply stop the treatment protocol altogether. Doing so can have adverse effects. Suddenly, such symptoms as mood swings, lethargy, weight gain, and fatigue begin to appear again. Sometimes the regression into an unhealthy state can be subtle—over a period of days or weeks—but sometimes it can be immediate. I do not chastise patients who are no longer following their programs. When you're finally feeling great, it's common to experience a sense of strength and stability and the feeling that you no longer need help. But in most cases, staying with treatment over the recommended period of time is critical in maintaining that balance for long periods of time.

Some of my patients will remain on treatment programs of one sort or another for the rest of their lives. But remember, our bodies' age and change constantly, so it's important that we pay attention to how we are feeling on an ongoing basis. Once we start to feel like our vital and youthful self again, our connection to our body is profound. We don't want to lose that sense of alignment, and we thus become extremely aware of how we're feeling.

It's also very important, particularly when you first get started in balancing your hormones, that you report to your doctor whether or not the desired improvements are taking place. Sometimes it takes a few adjustments in the treatment for improvements to occur. Even during the first few months, your body may change so dramatically that more extensive adjustments in dosages, supplements, and hormones have to be instituted. Everyone is unique. In integrative medicine, customizing treatment to your specific needs is essential.

The Art of Discovering What Is Truly Important in Your Life

We are born into this world as perfect, whole human beings with no knowledge of how humanity has created its systems and its rules. We spend a lifetime trying to fit in and continually trying to figure out exactly what our part is in this complicated, sometimes unforgiving world—a world that has been created by groups, nations, and a few key decision makers. Some of these confines are carefully developed to protect order in the world. However, some of these so-called values are used to control and manipulate people into becoming loyal consumers and invested believers. These "created" values may ultimately harm society as a whole.

For example, we spend an inordinate amount of time comparing ourselves to media images that, for all intents and purposes, we cannot possibly measure up to in real life. Even the models and actresses hired for these high-profile jobs have scars, imperfect skin, cellulite, extra weight, and more. Technology creates a fantasy version of these beautiful women that at times goes way beyond their own natural beauty. Those manipulated images are then presented to us as "reality." It takes an incredibly disciplined to dismiss those images as pure fiction. We end up wanting to be like these fictional images that eventually make us all feel inadequate.

Most of my patients are women, and it saddens me that so many of them do not have a consistent or prolonged sense of self-love. I would even go so far as to say that the typical self-images that I encounter are totally inconsistent with the beautiful, creative, intelligent, loving women I am privileged to care for. I encourage all the women in my life to stand back and to seriously question and reevaluate what happened in their lives to make them put themselves last. Was lack of self-love modeled by one or both parents? Were they unfairly ignored or criticized as children? Do they pay more attention to media images in magazines and on television than to the deeper spiritual truth that we are all divinely inspired creations? Do they look to others to feel a sense of self-worth, or can they tap into that sublime feeling of "all is well" in their own minds even during challenging times? Are they as forgiving and compassionate with themselves as they are with their loved ones? Perhaps they are angry all the time, because they do not feel accepted exactly as they are. And I wonder if they have an appropriate support system in place to deal with those feelings?

So much of these common feelings—lack of acceptance, discontent, and disassociation with our true selves—can be traced back to the moments in our lives when values were handed down to us under the guise of tradition or social expectations. If we looked a certain way, acted a certain way, or possessed certain things, we would be rewarded in this life with love and prosperity—enough of it to fill our days with joy, happiness, and security. But as we grow older, we should start to get a handle on the truth.

From a spiritual perspective, one of our primary mandates as human beings is to experience the ebb and flow of life so we can grow and become closer to the spirit within. Our lowest lows can become golden opportunities to reconnect with our true natures, which are built upon the profound universal principles of love, compassion, and joy. The more in alignment we are to living these core values that are present and possible in all human beings, the more happiness, health, and harmony can be ours. If we choose to operate from a place of love, compassion, and joy, it is impossible to harm ourselves or to harm others. We can live gracefully in a state of gratitude for what we have, and of forgiveness for those people and institutions who have, knowingly or unknowingly, tried to take us away from who we really are. We cannot always protect ourselves from the harshness of the world, and we cannot isolate our children fully from the overwhelmingly negative influences that our society heaps upon them from the time they are born. But what we can do is choose who we are with, how we spend our time, and what we allow ourselves to feel at any given moment. We can begin to release ourselves from the unreasonable expectations others put on us, and choose to live life *on our own terms.*

For many of my patients, even beginning the process of incorporating self-care into daily life is often viewed by family and friends as something silly, unnecessary, or selfish. This unfortunately, is a prevalent perception of self-care, as it can be viewed as a form of ego-centric behavior. That's how deep the urge to deny ourselves happiness can be. It is profound, even alarming, that we need to go through a process of consciously changing how we choose to care for ourselves. But the good news is that we are entering a new age of enlightenment that supports and promotes healthy lifestyles that go beyond working out and getting enough water. The concept of self-care is entering the mainstream at a rapid pace and will hopefully become part of a paradigm shift in the greater social consciousness so our children learn to find it quite strange when people do *not* take time to go for a walk, to enjoy a sunset, to create art for no reason other the pure joy of it, and to connect with people without the need for technology.

I would like to think that we're approaching an era where it's socially acceptable to take longer vacations, to prioritize fun, and to value relationships over material things. These are the natural values that emerge when people are honest about what they want in their lives. They want the freedom to be themselves, without judgment or admonishment. They want authentic and intimate relationships. They want clean organic food and purified water. They want creativity and the arts to be celebrated and cherished. They want to live harmoniously with the Earth and not against it. They want a deep, profound connection to a higher power. They want to do work that is personally meaningful and socially impactful. People ultimately seek a sense of peace, security, and joy. These realities come through allowing us to see, to acknowledge, and to experience that divine spark within. That spark is your connection to the universe, to spirit, to God—in whatever way is most comfortable to you. When someone is able to connect with that powerful and divine force within, health and healing become your natural state.

But let's be clear: the ego—those negative thoughts that demand that you eat that additional cupcake or urge you to yell back at that mean person—thrives on your insecurities and your past. It's the ego's job to keep you in a state of pain, confusion, and meltdown. The ego does not want you to live your divine truth—it wants you only to focus on your physical reality and the human part of your consciousness. The ego cannot stand it, not even for a second, when you make healthy physical and emotional choices. But the more often you make positive choices, the weaker the ego becomes, until eventually it is immobilized and put firmly in its place. We cannot deny this human part of ourselves. It is there to help us grow, to challenge us, and to create that necessary balance in our lives that promotes appreciation, strength, fortitude, and success. It's been said time and time again, that we cannot appreciate the beauty of flowers in the springtime if they also bloom in the winter. For everything, there is a season. Learning our core values are an important, even critical, step in reclaiming who we really are. That's the journey of a lifetime.

Medically speaking, we also need to be aware that we are simply not in charge of how our bodies function at all times. This is where the power of hormones makes itself profoundly obvious. When women come to me and proclaim, "I just don't feel like myself anymore," I feel very good knowing that I can reassure them in practical ways. Hormonal imbalances are responsible for a great deal of mood swings, fatigue, foggy thinking, depression and anxiety. It literally changes our brain chemistry. The United States is home to extraordinary research scientists and physicians who do nothing but study the relationship between hormones and the brain. Of course, the brain is the organ that helps us navigate through life, relationships, problems, creativity, and thinking in every way. This complex and powerful organ is the body's center of how we perceive ourselves and the world. It houses our personality, our values, and the way we manage experiences. So when hormones wreak havoc on brain chemistry, women report that they feel as though they have become entirely different people. And you can imagine what this does to daily life—relationships change, work patterns become more challenging, and the body begins to turn on itself through weight gain, hair loss, rapid aging, and more. For many women, these severe changes prompt depression, negative thinking, and spiritual crisis. Many women who come to me report experiencing a "dark night of the soul" where all seems lost. They cannot see that their brains are creating fertile and lush environments for their egos. They desperately want to become centered, compassionate, and spiritual once again, but the hormonal reality simply will not allow them to connect the all-important dots that create full and glorious pictures of their lives.

Without knowing the full repercussions of hormones gone wild, women put an incredible amount of pressure on themselves to change, to improve, and to just "get a handle" on their emotions. They don't understand why they are crying or screaming at the drop of a hat. They feel betrayed by their faiths. Adding insult to injury, they lack compassion from family and friends who honestly don't recognize the new personalities in the women they love. Furthermore, the changes seem like nature's cruel and heartless joke after a lifetime of devoting themselves to giving all they have and all they are to others. It doesn't seem at all fair that women can fall so far into the precocious hands of hormones at a time in their lives when they should be able to assert the most control in their lives. Women just want to live, to love, and to be who they are. And when hormones are under control, the opportunity to do that becomes a reality.

So what is important in your life? Before you begin to answer that question, I would highly recommend that you dig very deep and carefully consider what it is that you *truly* want in your life. Here are some questions to help you begin that important conversation with yourself:

I encourage you to answer the following questions to guide you on your personal journey to restoring your sense of true self through Health, Happiness, and Harmony:

1. What brings you joy on a daily basis?

_____

_____

_____

_____

_____

2. **What are the five most important aspects of your life?**

_____

_____

_____

_____

_____

3. **If money were not a consideration, how would you spend your time?**

_____

_____

_____

_____

_____

4. **If other people's opinions had no weight, would you conduct your life differently? If so, how?**

_____

_____

_____

_____

_____

5. **When you were a child, what made you happy? Do you still do those things as an adult? Why or why not?**

_____

_____

_____

_____

_____

6. *What are some talents and gifts that you had earlier in life that made you feel good about yourself?*

_____

_____

_____

_____

_____

7. *Do you find a sense of purpose and joy in helping other people? If yes, what do you want to do to help others?*

_____

_____

_____

_____

_____

8. *If this was your last day on Earth, what would you do, and who would you spend time with?*

_____

_____

_____

_____

_____

9. *In considering health, money, work, intelligence, spirituality, success, creativity, relationships, and love as the foundations of the human experience, how would you rank these in order of importance?*

_____

_____

_____

_____

_____

10. *If you could change 3 things about your life, what would they be?*

_____

_____

_____

_____

_____

11. *What is your bucket list? (Things you want to accomplish before you die?)*

_____

_____

_____

_____

_____

_____

_____

_____

_____

_____

_____

_____

_____

_____

_____

_____

_____

_____

_____

_____

CHAPTER 17:
STAYING TRUE TO YOURSELF

"There are only two ways to live your life.
One is as though nothing is a miracle.
The other is as though everything is a miracle"

ALBERT EINSTEIN

This final chapter focuses on keeping true to *yourself*. It does not focus on staying true to what your neighbors, kids, spouse, parents, society, media, other kids' moms, or anyone else thinks you should do or be. When you keep true to yourself, you create a pathway to light and love that can only bring peace, prosperity, and joy into your life and others' lives. And it's on this path that your friends and family can finally join you in a fulfilled and healthy life.

I am a spiritual woman, and I believe that God (or your Higher Power) wants the very best for each of us. We are mandated to care for ourselves in direct proportion to how much God (or your Higher Power) loves us. That's a tall order. But as human beings, we should try to embrace our humanness and connect to it daily with the spirit that lies ready and waiting to express the power of love, that is at our disposal at all times.

Firstly, we have to forgive ourselves for how we've abused our bodies or tolerated abuse from others. We have to do everything we can to trust in the divine universe, and not just the physical universe. Many faiths talk about realizing your true nature. It is a spiritual principle that suggests we all have the ability to reach enlightenment on Earth in human form. We don't have to wait until death to understand that we are all connected and part of one vast cosmic system. Our true nature is who we are when we forgive, celebrate, give thanks, express compassion, help, heal, and love. Our true nature was present when we were born and will be there when we die. Our true nature is immortal, and of the Divine Spirit. In fact, everyone's true nature is the same but expressed in personal and unique ways through mothering, creating, giving, loving, and even in receiving, from others. Although we all may have different personalities, family experiences, religious backgrounds, and challenges, the true nature of being human binds us. Finding our true nature and staying loyal to it day in and day out is our job as human beings. I have the privilege of seeing women transform before my eyes and return to who they really are through the power of physical and emotional healing.

I urge women to be gentle and deliberate in how they embark on their transformational journeys. Our tendency as women is to try to tackle every aspect of life all at once. When a woman makes up her mind to change her life, she usually develops a laundry list of to-dos—take a Pilates class, learn to meditate, volunteer at church, cook only organic food for the family, and more. We take our will to know our true natures and transform that urge into piles of action items, but that's not necessary. In fact, it's totally counter to the healing process. If your body, mind, and spirit are off track, chances are that some of those areas of your life need attention. Just start with one and them move to on to the others. Take it from there in a way that feels right to you. Be gentle with yourself. Love yourself truly and deeply. Cherish yourself as you would your own child. Honor yourself. Begin your journey with a positive feeling. Best of luck to you!

My Renewed Life Plan

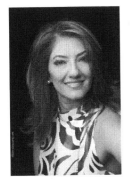

Dr. Shelena Lalji, also known as "Dr. Shel" by her patients and colleagues, is the founder and medical director of Dr. Shel Wellness & Medical Spa in Sugar Land, Texas. Her center is often referred to as the "Ultimate Destination for Beauty and Wellness". She has been inspiring and educating women on how to live their best lives possible by establishing a state of balance and harmony for well over 15 years.

Dr. Shel graduated from The Emory University School of Medicine and is a Board Certified Obstetrician and Gynecologist. After practicing traditional women's healthcare for over 13 years, she felt the need to focus on a comprehensive approach to women's wellness emphasizing the balance between the mind, body and spirit. This journey led her to establish her center, Dr. Shel Wellness & Medical Spa, in 2006 so that she could pass her inspiration on to her patients.

Her daily mission is to empower women to look and feel their best. She teaches them to cherish and honor themselves with her integrative knowledge and aesthetic treatments that combine the science of medicine and the art of beauty. She guides her patients through a journey consisting of natural, bio- identical hormones, nutrition, healthy living, state-of-the-art aesthetic procedures, and stress management strategies. She feels privileged to have empowered thousands of women, as well as to have educated countless practitioners about the benefits of a complete wellness approach.

Dr. Shel is the recipient of many awards, holds several volunteer positions and is a strong supporter of her community. She serves on the American Cancer Society Leadership Council, various Child Advocacy groups, Women's Shelter organizations, Women's Empowerment groups, Autism Support groups, and other causes that are dear to her heart. She is a sought after keynote speaker at numerous conferences including the Texas Conference for Women, the American Academy for Anti-Aging Medicine, Pri-Med Conferences, Aesthetic Conferences, Wellness Symposiums, and Laser Clinical Forums to name a few. Dr. Shel has appeared several times on many local and national television shows to help educate the public about healthy lifestyles, natural and alternative health approaches, aesthetics, and other women's issues.

She believes in and lives by a strong balance in her own life while enjoying and embracing her many roles as a physician, a woman's advocate, an educator, an entrepreneur, a wife and a mother of two beautiful children.

56472301R00109

Made in the USA
Columbia, SC
25 April 2019